The Complete Book of
Family Aromatherapy

foulsham

Bennett's Close, Cippenham, Berkshire, SL1 5AP

ISBN 0-572-01622-0

Copyright © 1993 Joan Radford

Photoset in Great Britain by Encounter Photosetting, Fleet, Hampshire
Printed in Great Britain by St. Edmundsbury Press Ltd.,
Bury St. Edmunds, Suffolk

THE COMPLETE BOOK OF
Family Aromatherapy

Joan Radford

foulsham

LONDON • NEW YORK • TORONTO • SYDNEY

Contents

Introduction   9

1. *Background to Aromatherapy*   13

2. *How Aromatherapy Heals*   24

3. *The Sense of Smell*   35

4. *Buying and Storing Your Oils*   43

5. *Cautionary Notes*   54

6. *Methods of Use*   60

7. *Getting to Know Essential Oils*   77

8. *Some Further Essential Oils*   105

9. *Massage for Everyone*   122

10. *Reflexology and Aromatherapy*   134

11. *Pregnancy and Afterwards*   141

12. *From Tots to Teens*   158

13. *Aromatherapy for Senior Citizens*   165

14. *Common Ailments and Conditions*   171

Suggested Reading   222

Reputable Suppliers   223

About the Author   224

DEDICATION

To Peter, with all my love. Also in loving memory of my dear friends Caroline Lindop and Lawrence Baine. My thanks to Bernie Hephrun, Pat Drummond, Ann Mathias, Pat Fuller and Eileen Lloyd for their help.

Introduction

AROMATHERAPY is the use of essential oils for their curative properties. An essential oil is a highly odiferous substance isolated from certain aromatic plants. The oil usually bears the name of the plant from which it is derived, for example jasmine or lavender, though there are a number of exceptions, such as neroli, which is extracted from orange blossom. In the plant the essence is stored as microdroplets in sacs or glands. According to the species, essential oil is obtained from the flowers, leaves, stems, roots, fruits or seeds, and sometimes from the whole plant. Even certain barks and woods are a source, yielding gums and resins from which the essential oil is extracted by distillation.

Essential oils are not greasy like the vegetable oils (e.g. olive, corn, soya). They are light, volatile, and made up of complex mixtures of organic chemicals (acids, esters, alcohols, aldehydes, ketones, terpenes and phenols).

Every essential oil used in aromatherapy has its own specific healing properties. Most of the oils are antiseptic to some degree, and will combat micro-organisms. A number of the oils can be used to calm the nervous system, others reduce inflammation, or ease aches and pains, benefit particular organs and systems of the body, uplift the spirits – the list could go on and on.

Some schools of aromatherapy advocate taking essential oils internally in certain circumstances. There is considerable controversy surrounding this. Personally, I think it is safer to make it a rule never to take any of them by mouth (gargles and mouthwashes are all right as they are not swallowed). Besides, external application and inhalation are usually considered faster and more effective methods of use than ingestion.

An important characteristic of essential oils is that they quickly penetrate the layers of the skin and enter the bloodstream. They are therefore fast-acting. But the oils are very strong and not generally applied undiluted to the skin. As they readily dissolve in fatty vegetable oils (not in water), they are conveniently used in massage oils, creams and lotions. (Clinical tests have shown that essential oils enter the bloodstream more quickly by inhalation than either through the skin or orally.)

Aromatherapy at Home

Using aromatherapy at home for yourself, your family and friends has considerable advantages. For a start, it will be cheaper than going for professional treatment, although the benefits of this should not be dismissed – there may still be times when you will want to consult a professional aromatherapist. Being able to carry out treatments at home is much more convenient than having to wait, sometimes several weeks, for an appointment with an aromatherapist. When you feel a symptom coming on, treatment can be immediate. The axiom 'prevention is better than cure' is a very good reason for such self-help.

You can do away with most of those proprietary medicines from the chemist – for coughs and colds, sinusitis, sore throats, headaches, and so on. Nor will you need to buy special skin creams, anti-cellulite lotions, air-fresheners, disinfectants and antiseptics.

The use of essential oils has a marked effect on the health of the skin. It would be blatantly dishonest for me to claim that aromatherapy can work miracles, reversing the ravages of time. However, I will state positively that essential oils can improve the tone and general condition of the skin and, if used regularly from about the age of 20, the effects of the ageing process can be delayed.

Unlike modern drugs and medicines, the essential oils in general use in aromatherapy rarely have unpleasant side effects. Instead, they help bring about harmony and well-being, peace and tranquillity. This book tells you how to use the different oils effectively and in complete safety.

In cases of anxiety, depression, tension and nervous excitability, essential oils are much safer than chemical tranquillisers and stimulants. The oils tend to be normalising or balancing rather than directly stimulating or sedating. Being of an organic, subtle nature, they act in similarly subtle and complex ways.

It takes a skilled professional aromatherapist to be able to select the best blend of oils for an individual. Not only will the therapist have a thorough knowledge of the effects of different oils on specific parts of the body, the psychological state of the client will be a major consideration too. A training course and experience gathered over years of practice of aromatherapy are necessary for anyone to acquire a high degree of expertise. But any person, with the aid of this book, can learn enough of the basics of aromatherapy to be able to tackle most minor disorders, injuries and psychological conditions. Knowing that one has an instant and effective remedy at hand is very comforting. I occasionally come across differing reactions to certain oils, but the well-tried formulas you'll find in Chapters 11 and 14 work well for most people.

Always be sensible with your health. If symptoms persist or you are not certain about their cause, consult a doctor. Orthodox medication does not interfere with the efficacy of aromatherapy treatments, or vice versa. Indeed, medical treatment and aromatherapy can help one another. Homoeopathic treatments, however, may be affected by certain aromatherapy oils (camphor, eucalyptus, peppermint).

Should you or a member of your family ever have major surgery or intense drug treatment for a serious illness, then stress and anxiety are likely to be felt on top of the discomforts of the treatment. During the recovery period, essential oils can help keep the sufferer calm and serene, relieve aches, pains and soreness and build up strength.

While essential oils are on the whole expensive, they do last for quite a long time. Your collection of oils can be built up gradually over a period of time until you have a nicely balanced and varied selection. On a non-therapeutic note, the oils may be used in the home for a wonderful way to enjoy your favourite flower aromas all the year round. An essence burner can create a garden atmosphere in a top-floor flat!

CHAPTER 1

Background to Aromatherapy

As LONG AGO as 4000 BC, the techniques of pressing, boiling and maceration were being used by civilisations in the East to obtain fragrant essences from flowers, leaves, woods, gums and resins. In the process of maceration, for example, the raw material would have been placed in warmed oil or fat and replaced with fresh batches, possibly as many as 15 times. The pomades and aromatic oils thus made were used in unguents (ointments) for annointing kings and holy men and for therapeutic purposes, cosmetics and perfumes.

The Egyptians and Babylonians used lavish amounts of perfumes and perfumed oils. Whilst animal fat was widely used for the basis of unguents, fatty oils were also used (extracted by cold pressing olives and the seeds of sesame, flax and the castor oil plant). Trade routes were established, for there was a lucrative market in spices, perfumes and incense.

Priests are considered to have been the first retailers of aromatics, dispensing them for perfume as well as for healing purposes. There was no distinction between holy perfumes and household perfumes. Some of the ingredients used then are still used today: frankincense, myrrh, galbanum (gum resins), cedarwood, sandalwood, cypress wood, lavender, camomile, marjoram, oregano, thyme, cinnamon, coriander, clove, roses, lilies, cornflower, jasmine and orange blossom.

The ancient Greeks and Romans also loved scented oils, unguents and pomades. These were so popular in the Roman Empire that quite a flourishing industry was set up. The rose was highly prized and used a great deal in perfumery, medicine, and even in food. Roses were tossed at the feet of homecoming Roman conquering armies, and handmaidens strewed rose petals at feasts. In Nero's golden palace, on special occasions the rooms were carpeted several inches deep in rose petals. The infamous Caligula believed in the therapeutic properties of aromatic baths to restore his body, exhausted by sexual excesses. Julius Caesar, however, did not think much of the highly perfumed Roman male – he'd prefer them to smell of garlic!

After the fall of the Roman Empire the use of perfumes and aromatics declined. But during the Middle Ages, the Arabian scientist, physician and philosopher Avicenna discovered (or perhaps rediscovered) the process of distillation for the extraction of rose oil and other plant essences. In fact his method was to be the basis of our modern distillation processes. Arabian perfumes soon became famous. The Crusaders brought aromatics back from the East to Europe, and before long a perfume industry developed in Europe itself.

Down the centuries mankind has relied mainly on plants for medicines. During the nineteenth and twentieth centuries, the science of chemistry developed enormously.

Drugs began to be created, and largely supplanted the old herbal medicines – though many modern drugs are still derived from plant sources (e.g. digitalis, from foxglove).

During the last 200 years technological advance in the production of essential oils has been considerable, as well as research into their chemistry. The term 'aromatherapy' was coined in 1937 by a French chemist, R.-M. Gattefossé. He had accidentally discovered the effectiveness of lavender oil on burns while working in a perfumery laboratory. In a small explosion he burned his hand and plunged it into the nearest liquid, which happened to be a bowl of lavender oil. The hand healed very quickly, with hardly a scar.

Subsequently, after researching into the beneficial properties of other essential oils, Gattefossé wrote: 'Doctors and chemists will be surprised at the range of odiferous substances which may be used medicinally and at the great variety of their chemical functions. Besides the antiseptic and antimicrobial properties of which use is currently made, the essential oils are also antitoxic and antiviral, they have a powerful energising effect and possess an undeniable cicatrising property. In the future their role will be even greater.'

That prophecy was to be fulfilled. A number of researchers and pioneers contributed their efforts. Notable among them was a French physician, Dr Jean Valnet, who was inspired by the work of Gattefossé. He used essential oils as antiseptics in the treatment of wounds in World War II. He also used the oils to combat tuberculosis, diabetes, cancer and other serious illnesses, claiming many successes. In 1964, Valnet published an important book on the subject, *Aromathérapie*.

Aromatherapy was greatly furthered by Marguerite

Maury, an Austrian biochemist and beautician. Since 1940 until the time of her death in 1968, she published two books, lectured on the subject throughout Europe, and opened aromatherapy centres in Paris, Switzerland and England. She ran courses giving information on the use of essential oils, with emphasis on their rejuvenating and cosmetic effects. Today we are used to the concept of healing holistically, i.e. taking the whole person into account and at all levels.

Well in advance, Marguerite Maury realised the importance of prescribing for the individual a mixture of oils that would restore balance, and not just on the physical level but on the mental and emotional levels too. She was also the first person to establish the technique of applying essential oils, diluted in vegetable oil, by massage.

Over the last 20 years there has been a tremendous upsurge of interest in the therapeutic uses of essential oils. Today, aromatherapy is accepted as a valued branch of complementary medicine and is still fast-growing in popularity.

Professional Treatment

Qualified aromatherapists treat clients for a variety of conditions, such as arthritis, circulatory problems, anxiety and depression, muscular stress and strain, migraines, menopausal troubles and rheumatism. The client is treated at a salon, clinic, private practice, or at home by a 'mobile therapist'.

If you consult an aromatherapist, initially you will be asked about your general health, eating and sleeping habits, amount of exercise and medical background. Then he or she will make up a blend of essential oils for massage. These will be the ones considered right for you as a whole person rather than just your symptoms. Many aromatherapists also use reflexology (treatment of specific ailments by foot massage) before a massage, as this helps pinpoint energy imbalance.

The results of aromatherapy treatment are usually seen after three or four sessions. Weekly or fortnightly sessions may be recommended to begin with, perhaps lessening to once a month. The improvement may be maintained by using the prescribed blend of oils at home. Clients may decide to have treatment once a week indefinitely, if they wish to maintain a permanent state of relaxation and well-being.

The massage relaxes both mind and body, relieving tension and anxiety. Unfortunately, many people wait until something goes wrong before they seek help. When aromatherapy treatments are kept up regularly (minimum once a month), all the systems are revitalised. This not only eliminates a good number of everyday problems but, in my opinion, helps to prevent major disease.

One of the benefits of visiting a therapist is the comfort factor. By this I mean the emotional support the client gets from human touch, and his/her relationship with the therapist – built on trust. He/she is able to unburden their problems without fear of criticism or judgement. Being able to talk about one's troubles in total confidence is one of the factors that promote health and well-being.

How Essential Oils are Obtained

All essential oils are volatile, a property which enables us to smell them; as they evaporate their vapours waft into our nostrils. Another characteristic of essential oils is that they are not heavy and greasy but generally have quite a watery consistency, though the viscosity does vary from type to type. The thicker ones include sandalwood and patchouli, but even these do not have the greasy texture of the vegetable oils extracted from seeds or nuts, such as sunflower, sesame and coconut.

Oils have a lower density than water – they float on top of it. Though essential oils are insoluble in water they will dissolve in alcohol and other organic liquids, and also in fats, waxes and other oils.

The above properties are utilised in the various extraction methods for obtaining essential oils.

Distillation

Most essential oils are obtained by distillation. The plant material, whatever it happens to be, is placed in a container and either boiled in water or subjected to steam under pressure. The heat causes the oil globules in the material to burst open. The released essence in the form of vapour, together with steam, then passes through a condenser where water cooling takes place. Here the vapours turn back into liquids which are collected in a flask. The essential oil floats on top of the condensed water and is therefore easily run off.

Solvent extraction

The strong heat and pressure used in the distillation process just described would damage the oil of some flowers, notably rose, jasmine and orange blossom. In these cases a different method can be used. One of these is called solvent extraction. The essential oil dissolves in the solvent liquid as it flows slowly over the petals. The solvent is then distilled off at a low temperature. The product, which still contains some waxes, is a semi-solid called a 'concrete'. When this is shaken in alcohol the waxes are removed, leaving a high quality flower oil (an 'absolute').

In the past, the solvents used in the solvent extraction process would have been liquids such as alcohols, petroleum and ether. Today, liquid butane or carbon dioxide may be used, producing very high quality oils.

Enfleurage

The oldest method of extracting essential oils is called enfleurage, in which the flower essence is absorbed by fat. Sheets of glass are coated with the fat, lard for example, over which fresh flowers are sprinkled. The coated glass is then stacked in tiers for many days, during which time the essences are absorbed by the fat. As the flowers deteriorate they are replaced by new ones. Finally saturation point is reached and the fat is collected. The essence-infused fat (now called a pomade) is shaken in alcohol for many hours to separate off the essence. An alternative though similar method uses sheets of muslin stretched over wooden frames and soaked in olive oil. Both these traditional methods, which have been used in the perfume industry, produce very high quality oils. However, they are time consuming and the product is therefore very expensive.

Enfleurage is no longer used commercially except to produce oil of tuberose, which is worth its weight in gold. The world's total yearly production of tuberose oil is only about 15 kilograms. Cultivated in France and Morocco, the blossoms are hand-picked, wrapped in damp cloths and extracted with lard as outlined above. Tuberose, as far as I'm aware, is not used for aromatherapy – heaven forbid at the price! It is only used in the most expensive perfumes.

Absolutes

The high-quality oils that are the end-product of solvent extraction or enfleurage are termed *absolutes*. Strictly speaking, only the oils extracted by distillation should be called essential oils. From the point of view of aromatherapy, there is a difference between absolutes and oils obtained by distillation. The former have a stronger perfume and a greater therapeutic power and hence should be used in lower concentrations. Also, they have a thicker consistency and tend to be coloured.

Expression method

The aromatic oils of citrus fruits can be obtained simply by the application of pressure – a method known as expression. Originally the rind of the fruit was squeezed by hand into a sponge to collect the oil. Although the best quality citrus oils are still extracted by hand, machinery is more often used today. The peel is ruptured and the 'cold pressed' grades of orange, lemon, bergamot, mandarin, grapefruit and lime oils are obtained. Lime oil can also be distilled but the aroma produced in this instance is different.

Because the demand for citrus oils has increased, fruit juice manufacturers have been producing cheaper citrus oils as side products. After the fruit is separated from the pith, it is pulped with the rind to extract the juice. The pulp is then distilled to produce essential oils from the vapour.

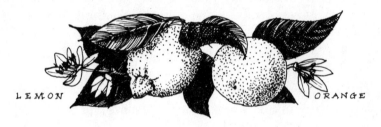

Factors Affecting Composition

The composition of an essential oil can vary quite considerably according to where the plant is grown. Basil, a plant belonging to the Labiatae family, produces an oil containing an organic compound called methyl chavicol. The proportion of this substance in basil grown in the Comoro Islands is 80%, whereas basil from Egypt (sometimes called French basil) yields approximately 25%.

Other factors causing variations in the chemical character of specific oils are the particular strain or variety of plant used, the climate in which the plant is grown, the method of agriculture (notably the use or not of pesticides and chemical fertilisers), the soil type and altitude. For example, lavender grown at high altitude produces an oil with a higher ester (linalyl acetate) content, giving it a higher odour quality.

Natural Versus Synthetic

Think of everything in your home that has a flavour or scent: bottles of perfume and toilet water, soap, shampoo, talcum powder, bath salts, lemon-scented washing up liquid, fabric conditioner, floor polish (the list is endless). These products all contain aromatic substances, some of which may be essential oils. Some ingredients, though, will be synthetic, that is, produced in a factory and not by a plant.

Let us consider modern perfumes. These generally contain only about 15 per cent natural ingredients, because of the high cost. Very expensive perfumes are likely to contain natural rose oil, but even then the quantity present would only be in the region of 1 per cent.

Many aromatic substances in commercial use are man-made and rightly so. After all, who needs pure unadulterated essence of pine in a floor-cleaning liquid? Essential oils for use in therapy, however, must be of the finest quality. They should contain neither additives nor chemical extenders as these can damage delicate tissues and, furthermore, are likely to be absorbed by the skin and into the body where harm can be done.

Most plant essences have an extremely complex chemical make-up. They consist of a number of different organic compounds, i.e. they all contain the element carbon, together with other elements (mainly hydrogen and oxygen). The most common groups of compounds in essential oils are the terpenes, camphenes, derivatives of the phenols and benzene, alcohols, aldehydes and esters, geraniol and linalool. But plant chemistry is for the boffins; we don't need to wrestle with it in order to practice aromatherapy at home.

Chemists are apparently able to analyse the various constituents of a particular oil and combine the separate ingredients in the correct proportions to produce that oil artificially – this can be cheaper than extracting the natural oil. Consider natural rose oil, for example. Perfume chemists know that it contains about 500 substances (the majority of which are present in minute proportions). However, they are getting close to being able to recreate a rose oil that smells just like the natural kind. Whilst reconstituted oils have a place in the perfume industry, their therapeutic potency is usually found to be inferior to that of the natural oils. Why is this so?

There is something about the way natural oils are constructed that chemists have not been able to discover. They cannot reproduce them properly by artificial means – only nature can do that, through the vital energy, the dynamic forces found in living things. Perhaps these same dynamic forces have something to do with the healing power of the plant and its essences.

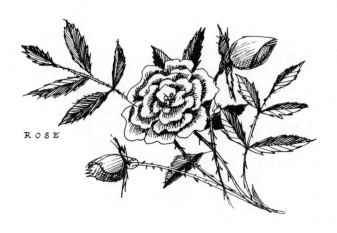

ROSE

CHAPTER 2

How Aromatherapy Heals

FROM THE VERY EARLIEST TIMES, people have been making use of the beneficial and curative effects of plants. For primitive man, finding out which plants have healing properties may have been, initially, a matter of trial and error; perhaps instinct played a part. Once gained, the knowledge would have been passed on verbally.

Eventually mankind learned to write, and hundreds of years ago the first herbals – books about herbs – were written. The medicines described in them were mainly aqueous extractions. These were made by either pouring water over the herb and steeping it, or by simmering it, and then straining before drinking. Poultices were the hot application of the herb itself. Ointments would be made by placing the herb into lard until it was saturated with the properties of the herb, then the fat would be melted and run off into jars to cool.

Today, a large number of people are turning to herbal therapy as a more natural, safe form of treatment for their ailments than pharmaceuticals. Unlike our forebears, however, who would have gathered fresh herbs to make infusions and decoctions – usually nasty tasting – the tendency is to purchase packaged pills that are quick and easy to swallow. One can also purchase ready-made tinctures, lotions and ointments for external use.

Active Principals and Properties

Medicinal plants contain active principles, i.e. compounds that act upon the organism. Some of these compounds have been isolated and are used in modern medicines and drugs, e.g. atropine from deadly nightshade *(Atropa bella-donna)*. Of course many of the medicinal plants are extremely poisonous, as in this example, and are not for use in the home. The fact that a substance comes from a plant does not mean it has no dangerous side effects. There are essential oils, too, which, if used in large amounts and/or too frequently can do serious harm (see pp. 58–59).

The properties of specific medicines are divided into categories according to their physiological effects. For example, a certain medicine or preparation may be described as analgesic (pain-relieving), or carminative (expels wind), and so on. Specific essential oils can be classified in the same way.

Properties of some popular essential oils

ANALGESIC

Pain relieving: bergamot, cajuput, camomile, lavender, peppermint, rosemary, tea-tree.

ANTIDEPRESSANT

Helps to lift depression: basil (Egyptian), bergamot, camomile, clary sage, geranium, jasmine, lavender, melissa, neroli, orange, patchouli, rose, sandalwood, ylang ylang.

ANTI-INFLAMMATORY

Reduces inflammation: cajuput, camomile, lavender, peppermint, rose.

ANTISEPTIC

Kills micro-organisms. Most essential oils are antiseptic to a degree. The following are markedly antiseptic: bergamot, eucalyptus, juniper berry, lavender, lemon, lemongrass, orange (sweet), pine, rosemary, sandalwood, tea-tree, thyme.

ANTISPASMODIC

Relieves muscle spasm/cramp: black pepper, cajuput, camomile, clary sage, eucalyptus, fennel, juniper berry, lavender, marjoram, orange (sweet), rose, rosemary.

APHRODISIAC

Reputed to increase sexual desire: clary sage, fennel, jasmine, neroli, patchouli, rose, rosemary, sandalwood, ylang ylang.

ASTRINGENT

Contracts tissues and reduces the flow of secretions and discharges: cedarwood, cypress, frankincense, geranium, lemon, myrrh, patchouli, rose, sage, sandalwood.

CARMINATIVE

Relieves flatulence: camomile, cardamom, clove, fennel, ginger, peppermint, spearmint.

CICATRISANT

Stimulating the formation of scar tissue: frankincense, lavender, neroli, rose, sandalwood.

DEODORANT

Combats body odour: citronella, cypress, eucalyptus, lavender, rosemary, tea-tree.

DIURETIC

Promotes the flow of urine: cedarwood, cypress, fennel, geranium, grapefruit, juniper berry, lavender, lemon, patchouli, sage.

EMMENAGOGUE

Induces or stimulates the menstrual flow: basil (Egyptian), camomile, clary sage, fennel, hyssop, lavender, marjoram, rose, rosemary, sage (Spanish).

EXPECTORANT

Facilitates the break-up of catarrh: basil (Egyptian), bergamot, cedarwood, eucalyptus, fennel, hyssop, lavender, lemon, sage (Spanish), sandalwood.

FUNGICIDAL

Inhibits the growth of microscopic fungi: tea-tree.

HEPATIC

Liver tonics: camomile, cardamom, lemon, peppermint, rose.

HYPERTENSIVE

Raises low blood pressure: rosemary.

HYPOTENSIVE

Reduces high blood pressure: geranium, lavender, lemon, melissa, ylang ylang.

NERVINE

Tonics for nervous disorders: basil (Egyptian), bay, bergamot, camomile, clary sage, cypress, geranium, jasmine, lavender, lemon, mandarin, marjoram, melissa, neroli, orange, patchouli, peppermint, rose, sage (Spanish), sandalwood. For nervines with a mainly calming effect, see Sedative.

RUBEFACIENT

Stimulates peripheral blood supply: black pepper, cajuput, coriander, eucalyptus, ginger, juniper berry, rosemary.

SEDATIVE

Nervines that predominantly calm and soothe: camomile, clary sage, myrrh, marjoram, neroli, sandalwood, ylang ylang.

STIMULANT

Excites and increases physical or mental function. Circulatory: black pepper, geranium, rose, rosemary, thyme. Mental: basil (Egyptian), eucalyptus, lemon, lemongrass, peppermint, tea-tree, thyme.

TONIC

Strengthens the whole system, increasing a feeling of well-being: basil (Egyptian), frankincense, geranium, lemon, melissa, myrrh, rose, sandalwood.

What is Special about Aromatherapy?

How is it that tiny amounts of essential oils, absorbed into the bloodstream and tissues via the skin, can have marked therapeutic benefits, both physically and mentally?

One possible explanation is that some molecules in essential oils act like hormones; these may form a relationship with the our own hormones, travelling through the body systems, revitalising and regulating our emotional and physical responses. Essential oils appear also to stimulate the body's defences against infection. Some essences are more effective than others in this respect, e.g. tea-tree. They appear to work through their power to promote the formation of the white corpuscles in the blood that attack harmful microbes.

It has been found that certain essential oils have an affinity for particular organs of the body, e.g. lavender with the kidneys, cypress with the ovaries. It would seem that if an organ is sluggish it will selectively absorb a substance that can boost its action just like it would absorb a nutrient. Dr Valnet suggested that geranium, pine, rosemary and sage stimulate the adrenal cortex (an endocrine gland) and alleviate tension caused by stress. And similarly, mint stimulates the pituitary cortex which affects most of the other hormone-producing glands.

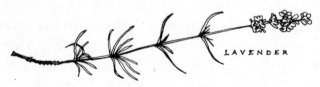

LAVENDER

Calming effects of essential oils

As we all know, the mind, emotions and physical body interact. Glands, blood vessels, heart, lungs and intestines are regulated by the autonomic nervous system which in turn is affected by the state of our mind. Prolonged stress or anxiety can lead to various physical disorders. Overstimulation of gastric juices, for example, may give rise to peptic ulcer.

Apart from the tension-relieving effect mentioned on page 30, the mind and emotions may be soothed by essential oils in other ways. For example, an oil may have a direct sedative or stimulating effect on the nerves. In particular, the very perception of a pleasant fragrance can have a soothing, uplifting effect, dispelling depression.

Different odours, nice, nasty or indifferent, affect our moods in various ways. The nerve pathways associated with the sense of smell are in very close proximity to the brain. They connect with a part of the brain known as the limbic system, which is responsible for our feelings and emotions. This is largely why the aromas of essential oils can have such an influence on our moods and feelings. We will pursue the subject of the sense of smell more fully in the next chapter.

When using essential oils you are likely to notice that some of them have both a stimulating and a sedative effect. This seems like a contradiction but it is not. Supposing you wish to be calmed and soothed but not be drowsy as you need to continue with work. One of the following oils would be a good choice: basil, bergamot, grapefruit, lavender, sandalwood. On the other hand, if you want to relax totally to the point of being soporific, you could choose a sedative oil such as camomile, clary sage or jasmine.

How aromatherapy differs from herbal medicine

Although aromatherapy is allied to herbal medicine in that they are both based on substances derived from plants, there are distinct differences. The properties of an extracted plant essence are not likely to be exactly the same as those of a herbal infusion or decoction, albeit from the same kind of plant. The preparation techniques are different, and these have a bearing on the chemical constituents, and therefore the properties, of the end-product. Heat is usually employed both in the production of herbal extracts, i.e. those used as medicines, and in the extraction of essential oils. Boiling can destroy some ingredients but, on the other hand, some volatile oils need a sustained high temperature to permit extraction.

The very process of distillation can alter the constituents of an oil. A very good case in point is the essential oil of camomile. This contains a blue-violet crystalline substance called azulene. Azulene is not present in the fresh flower but is formed when the oils are distilled. Azulene is a healing agent in skin conditions (see p. 80).

There is some evidence that when a known active constituent is present in an essential oil, its properties may be found to be greater than when it has been isolated and used alone for treatment. A possible explanation is that the minor constituents of the oil contribute in a major way to its therapeutic properties (as well as to its colour and odour). To give an example, it has been demonstrated that the essential oil of eucalyptus has greater antiseptic properties than isolated eucalyptol, its principal constituent. An analogy may be made here with vitamins. It is now widely recognised that other substances have to be present with a vitamin for it to be fully utilised in the body. Vitamin C is a good case in point. Its action is helped by the substances known as bioflavonoids, which always accompany the vitamin in foods and are sometimes included in vitamin C tablets.

When isolated, some constituents of essential oils can have an irritant effect on the skin, though when the rest of the constituents of the natural oil are present no skin reaction occurs. An example of this is oil of lemongrass, which contains citral, an aldehyde that will cause a skin reaction if used in isolation. (Some essential oils are toxic, and of course these are not used in aromatherapy.)

Many aromatherapists claim that the therapeutic properties of essential oils tend to be greater in combination than when used alone – the components are said to be working synergistically. I am not wholly convinced that this is so, though blending is useful in that one can combine several therapeutic properties in one treatment as well as creating delightful aromas.

Some further aspects of healing

An important part of aromatherapy is massage, which encourages absorption of oils into the skin and stimulates the circulation (see Chapter 9). The caring human touch and the ability to be able to talk about personal problems without fear of criticism can aid the healing process.

A good aromatherapist will take into consideration the

whole person and not just the ailing part or symptom. The subject of 'holistic' healing is too deep and involved to be dealt with adequately here, but its basic principles can be mentioned. If you are ill and in pain, a practitioner would treat the symptom first to relieve the discomfort. A holistic practitioner would also, in the longer term, treat the fundamental cause in an effort to prevent the problem recurring. Not only the body but the mind and spirit needs to be taken into account. A balance needs to be brought about within the whole self for health, well-being, inner peace and tranquillity. Aromatherapy is an ideal means towards achieving this.

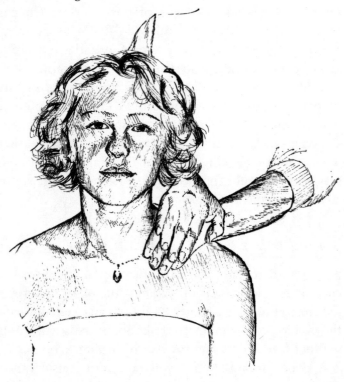

CHAPTER 3

The Sense of Smell

WE ARE CAPABLE of recognising 4000 different scents, and a highly sensitive nose might be able to identify as many as 10,000. When somebody is blind and deaf, the enormous potential of the sense of smell compensates for the loss of hearing and sight.

How do we smell something? Here is a very brief summary. Specialised cells in the nasal cavity receive stimuli from the airborne odour particles, olfactory nerves transmit the stimuli to the brain where the signals are passed along the olfactory tract to several brain areas, and nerve cells in the temporal lobes of the cerebrum (part of the fore-brain) interpret the stimuli.

It is worth looking into the process in more detail.

In the upper part of the mucus membrane of the nasal cavities, on each side, is a little patch of receptor cells. Although each of these olfactory membranes is not much larger than a thumbnail, together they contain approximately 20 million receptor cells. Projecting from each cell are eight or more fibrils which identify the scent. Odour molecules reaching the receptor cells stimulate them to send rapid impulses through adjoining nerve fibres.

These nerve fibres from the receptor cells pass through tiny apertures in a wafer-thin section of bone called the

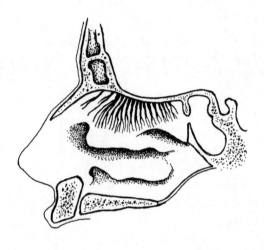

Filaments of the olfactory nerves

cribriform plate which is at the front of the cranial cavity. The nerve fibres run directly into an outlying portion of the brain called the *olfactory bulbs* (there are two). No bigger than match heads, the bulbs are located just behind the bridge of the nose and about 1 cm into the head. From this region, sensations are passed along a web of nerve tracts into many parts of the brain.

Most of the nerve pathways associated with smell terminate in the central regions of the brain thought to have been the earliest to develop during the course of evolution. These are the parts mostly responsible for our basic emotions and sexual behaviour. There are further connections with the pituitary gland, the master gland of the endocrine system. Some connections, of course, are made with the outer part of the brain (the cortex). This region of the brain developed later on, and is responsible for higher thought processes.

Thoughts and feelings interact with one another. Some scientists go so far as to assert that all our emotions are the result of neurochemicals and hormones released into the bloodstream. Be that as it may, essential oils are widely believed to stimulate or normalise the release of hormones and neurochemicals in the body (massage is also said to bring this about). This could explain why aromatherapy brings about a state of well-being.

It has also been claimed that essential oils themselves act like hormones in the body, stimulating glandular secretions. Whether this is so or not, one can at least say that the effect of the essences on the emotions and on the nervous system suggests an influence on the endocrine system. Fennel oil is known to contain a form of the hormone oestrogen. For this reason it is often used to treat menstrual disorders, but it should be avoided in pregnancy.

Some aromas can trigger the release of memories, either pleasant or unpleasant.

Through the effects that certain essential oils have upon our senses they can help us to clarify our thoughts, be more aware of ourselves (and others) and act more positively.

Scientists have begun to unravel the complex hormonal and neurological avenues relating to smell. They now predict that in the future it will be possible to manipulate mood, emotions and behaviour by using the right scents (to some extent, that is what aromatherapists have been doing for some while). A recent report on scientific research into the use of aroma says that, although it sounds like 'science fiction', aromas were being formulated that could stimulate or calm people. It was also suggested that directors of large companies should give a quick spray of an 'aroma activate' before summoning executives for important board meetings.

Today, some hospitals and surgeries use citrus or woody smells to allay patients' fears. And office workers have been exposed to specific aromas to increase their alertness (an essence burner on every desk). Computer workers in Japan performed more efficiently after their working environment was scented with lemon.

Warwick University experts developed an aroma reminiscent of the seaside. It was believed to be a blend of seaweed aroma, woody fragrances and sun lotion. This was used experimentally in the treatment of severe chronic anxiety and agoraphobia (fear of open spaces).

The scientists still have some mysteries to solve relating to the sense of smell. Although they have been able to demonstrate that in the sense of taste – to which smell is closely related – there are four primary flavours, sweet, sour, bitter and salt, they have not been as successful in classifying smells. Some say there are seven basic odours, others say there are 50 or more, and still others maintain that every odour is a primary one.

The Art of Smelling Essential Oils

Most people's sense of smell is underdeveloped and needs to be trained. So, before launching into the practical techniques of aromatherapy, let's begin with some experiments that will enhance your powers of distinguishing aromas.

First of all, obtain at least four essential oils, but no more than six. More than this will confuse your nose and eventually you will not be able to differentiate between the odours. Cedarwood will smell like lavender and lavender like rosemary. (Lemongrass will always smell like lemongrass!)

Next, choose an area away from other strong aromas (kitchens, etc.). The temperature of the room should be warm and it should be free from draughts. Breathe in and out quite quickly through your nose in order to clear the nasal passages.

Write the name of each essential oil you are going to test on coffee filter papers or strips of blotting paper. Test one oil at a time. Dip the end of the strip – about ½ inch – into the oil. Then hold the paper just under your nose – about ½–1 inch away – avoiding touching the skin.

When I am conducting a lesson on essences, I ask my students to write down their impressions of the aroma. As well as a describing the quality of the aroma, they record the mental effect it has on them, for example, sedative, stimulating, uplifting, refreshing.

Aromas are usually defined in 'notes'.

Top note: This is the characteristic first impression. Top notes are sharpish, evaporate quickly, and usually last 20–30 minutes.

Middle note: This is classed as the heart or bouquet and fully develops between 1 and 2 hours, sometimes longer. It lasts for a day or two.

Base note: The bottom note is the heaviest, gives an aroma its strength and is the last to go.

These notes sometimes overlap, i.e. you may find a base note that will also show a middle note and a middle note showing a top note.

Try the following experiment. Pour a few drops of different essential oils onto separate pieces of blotting paper and smell them at intervals. Which ones are the first to fade? Does the aroma alter after a time? Oils that have a predominant top note include bergamot, eucalyptus, lemon, tea-tree. Oils with a distinctive base note include frankincense, sandalwood and ylang ylang. Somewhere in the middle you will find camomile, fennel and geranium. These are just a few examples.

The following terms are used to describe the aromas:

BALSAMIC 🌸 warm and sweet with a soft odour of resins.

CAMPHORACEOUS 🌸 clean and medicinal, such as camphor.

HERBACEOUS 🌸 having a distinct odour of herbs or garden plants.

METALLIC 🌸 cold steel, cool and clear.

GREEN 🌸 fresh and grasslike.

SPICY 🌸 having an aroma reminiscent of cinnamon or nutmeg, warm.

WOODY 🌸 a warm, leaflike aroma more than a definite wood tone.

FRUITY 🌸 having an aroma of fruit (apples, pears, etc.).

FLORAL 🌸 usually a sweet aroma, smelling of flowers.

SWEET 🌸 an aroma like vanilla, peach or jam.

CITRUS 🌸 fresh tangy orange, lemon or lime tones.

Try describing a few essential oils using the above terms. Record the aroma after 15 minutes, 30 minutes, 2 hours, 1 day, 1 week. The examples below will serve as a guide –

GERANIUM

Top note: Powerful, sweet, honey-like, rosy odour with minty fresh undertones.

Middle note: Still minty – rose tone deepens.

Base note: Still a trace of mintiness – rose tone is slightly peppery and metallic.

EUCALYPTUS

Top note: Pungent, refreshing, camphoraceous, head-clearing.

Middle note: Slightly woody tone.

Base note: Non-existent

ROSE ABSOLUTE

Top note: Rich and rosy, like tea with honey, soft and floral.

Middle note: Richer honey tones, still rosy.

Base note: Still rosy in character – honey not as sweet.

YLANG YLANG

Top note: Warm, floral, slightly medicinal – the better quality oil is very like jasmine.

Middle note: Floral tone develops – warmer.

Base note: More like jasmine – still rich and floral.

Make your own blends

Having trained your nose you should find no difficulty blending oils together to achieve really satisfying aromas. You will find out which oils tend to be overpowering in a blend and are best used in tiny amounts. In a good blend the components will complement each other. For example, try sharp, sweet oils such as citrus (lemon, mandarin, sweet orange, grapefruit) with warm, spicy ones such as ginger, coriander, cardamom. The soft woody tone of sandalwood blends well with a floral type, such as geranium, rose or ylang ylang.

CHAPTER 4

Buying and Storing Your Oils

MOST ESSENTIAL OILS will remain effective for up to two years, provided they are kept in suitable containers. They are usually supplied in dark glass bottles – amber, dark green or blue. If you change the container, make sure you label it clearly. When mixing blends, keep them in similar glass bottles, which you can buy from a chemist. Plastic bottles cannot be used as containers for more than eight weeks as the oils will deteriorate.

The vegetable oils used as a base for essential oils will not hold the aroma or properties of the essence for very long; without preservatives the vegetable oil will oxidise it, resulting in loss of effectiveness. For this reason, I suggest not making up more than 100 ml at any one time.

Store your oils in a cool place out of direct sunlight and away from naked flames. As essential oils are volatile, make sure the bottle top is always properly secured.

Keep essential oils away from children. Do not keep them in any bottle or location where they could be mistaken for medicines or drinks.

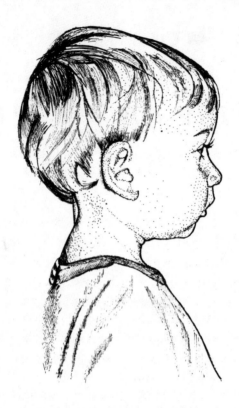

Keep essential oils away from children

Purchasing Essential Oils

It is advisable to find a reputable supplier because descriptions in sales literature cannot always be relied upon. If you have any difficulty, I can vouch for the purity and quality of the oils marketed by the mail order companies whose details are given on p. 223.

By means of highly sensitive chemical tests – gas chromatography – it is possible for companies to find out whether the oils sent to them by suppliers are indeed unadulterated and of a purity essential for use in aromatherapy. The colour of particular oils may vary a little from time to time. But if you find that all the essential oils you have purchased are colourless, there is a problem somewhere!

Availability and price of essential oils

Generally speaking, the cost of a particular oil is higher the lower the yield per kilo of plant material used in its production. There are exceptions, however. Lavender yields quite a low percentage of essential oil per load (1.6 % approx.) but the oil is relatively inexpensive (about £3.50 per 10 ml bottle at the time of writing). This is because lavender is widely cultivated; literally fields and fields of it are grown in many countries of the world, and therefore it is available in large quantities. Also, lavender doesn't need fertilisers or pesticides (see p. 46).

Frankincense and myrrh yield quite a large percentage of oil from the gum resin but they are quite expensive in comparison with lavender (about £10.00 per 10 ml bottle). The trees grow wild and crops are comparatively scarce. Sandalwood, again fairly pricey, is not considered oil-producing until the trees are 25–30 years old.

Details of the most popular and useful essential oils are given in Chapters 7 and 8.

Organically grown oils

The fashion now is for 'organic' oils. All living plants are organic, of course. The usual definition of 'organically grown' is that the plants are produced in conformity with the strict guidelines set down by the Soil Association. It takes five years or more for soil to become free of chemicals; therefore if plants are not sprayed with chemicals but grown in unclean soil they are not strictly 'organic'. If you see any product sold as 'organic' that does not carry the Soil Association's symbol, the seller should be challenged.

Overseas, producers and sellers of organically grown produce come under the umbrella of the International Federation of Organic Agricultural Movement (IFOAM). Eventually EEC regulations will make it illegal to sell products as organically grown unless they carry the EEC organic symbol or that of the designated governmental body which in the United Kingdom is the Soil Association.

Meanwhile, certain companies are making extraordinary claims in this field. At present there are very few organically grown essential oils on the market, and since they are only available in very small quantities they command a high price. Lavender is one of the exceptions. The plant produces its own insecticide, so it doesn't need to be sprayed with chemicals. It will also grow on poor soils and therefore doesn't require the application of fertilisers. The oil is naturally organic.

'Pure' (and 'pure organic') oils

An essential oil described as 'pure' should not have been mixed or diluted with any other substance. Ideally it should be free from tainting or polluting matter. Nevertheless, it would not be quite accurate to state that it is 100 per cent pure because almost certainly there will be impurities present, i.e. traces of substances from the soil in which the plant grew and possibly also air pollutants.

Ideally, all essential oils for use in aromatherapy should be organically grown and distilled with care. Growers and producers are likely to become increasingly more aware of this need as the popularity of aromatherapy grows.

'Natural' oils

This description means existing in or produced by nature. Strictly speaking, only those essential oils obtained from plants grown in the wild can be called 'natural'. But the plants mainly used nowadays in the production of essential oils are specially cultivated for the purpose. They are propagated by taking cuttings and grafting, which again is not 'natural'.

'True' oils

This word is being used to define essential oils. It means factually accurate, not false, fictional or illusory. But what does the retailer mean by 'true'. True to botanical source, purity and nature? Or true, it was man-made in a laboratory? 'True' certainly sounds nice, and reputable companies will use this adjective for all the right reasons. The problem is, relatively unknown companies with no established credentials are describing their wares as 'pure and natural true organic oils'!

In the early days, companies selling essential oils (mine

included) were all guilty of labelling our goods as 100 per cent pure/natural/unadulterated. Now I believe the companies with integrity have dropped the hype and are relying on their reputation, knowledge and understanding of essential oils; they use expressions such as top or high quality (general excellence).

Watch out for adulteration

So-called 'nature identicals' are substances produced chemically for the perfume industry. These can be used to adulterate or even 'make' essential oils for the unsuspecting supplier. Another method of adulteration is to extend or 'cut' with a chemical substance or with terpenes removed from other essential oils. You have to know your supplier very well and trust him or send your oils away for analysis (hardly practical).

The greatest problem is the supplier who knows little about essential oils. I have been astounded at the blatant adulteration of essential oils in some retail outlets. I remember going into a craft shop recently where, among the pot pourri, scented candles and suchlike, there was a display of '100 per cent pure essential oils for aromatherapy'. My curiosity got the better of me and I started testing them. They were dreadful, obviously not from any natural botanical source. The viscosity was wrong and my nose smelt a rat (figuratively of course). One of the first signs that told me they were not pure was the price. Sandalwood, jasmine and neroli were all priced at £2.95 for 25 ml. When I challenged the shopkeepers, a young couple, they assured me that the oils were indeed 100 per cent pure. I asked them how they could be sure and whether they knew anything about aromatherapy.

They both looked rather shocked and sheepish, saying their supplier had told them the oils were pure.

'Aromatherapy oils'

The public can be misled by products described as 'aromatherapy oils'. These are essential oils that have been put into a vegetable or mineral oil. It is not an adulteration if the literature on the bottle states clearly that it is a blended oil ready for application. If, on the other hand, it is sold as essential oil it would be classified as adulterated.

This can be an excellent way of buying the more expensive oils (rose, neroli and jasmine), provided of course the essential oils are genuine. Market intelligence on suppliers is not easy to come by. Ask questions and study the literature of the seller. Use your intuition and start to train your nose. If a company appears to be selling oils all at the same price or too cheaply, buyer beware!

Signs to look for

If you have tried the exercises for training one's nose (pp. 39–42), you will easily be able to carry out the following test. Drop a little of the suspicious oil onto a piece of blotting paper. If the aroma disappears too quickly adulteration is likely – probably with alcohol.

Now test the texture. If it is oily and spreads either on paper or on your skin, it has had an oil of vegetable origin added to it. Oils that are extended leave an oily residue.

We know that essential oils have a shelf life and are usually stored in amber or dark brown bottles. If an oil is sold in a clear glass bottle, be suspicious.

Bases

Vegetable oils are used in aromatherapy massage blends. They serve to dilute the essential oils, which are too strong to be applied direct to the skin. The base oil also acts as a lubricant for the hands during massage.

If you dislike the feel of oil on the skin, an alternative is to use a white lotion base. Several mail order companies supply lotion bases, including the ones named on p. 223.

Purchasing base oils

When choosing base oils for your massage blends, my advice again is to buy only top quality even though it costs more. The best vegetable oils are cold-pressed from the first pressing, i.e. extra virgin. In later extractions, heat and solvents are used.

Avoid mineral oils as bases as they have little penetrating power. They stay on the surface of the skin and impede the absorption of essential oils. Furthermore, mineral oils have a drying effect with prolonged use. Baby oil, incidentally, is sometimes mineral based and may contain synthetic perfumes.

Choosing your base

There are a number of vegetable oils widely used as bases. They all have their own characteristics and special uses. It is worth remembering that some vegetable oils are nourishing for dry and ageing skin, and several contain useful amounts of minerals and vitamins. Vitamin E oil can be added to any base oil to improve dry skin.

The lighter oils are the best all-purpose carriers. Some of the vegetable oils that are rich in vitamin E are also rather thick and sticky; they need to be blended with less viscous oils (at 10–20%). Any oil you wish to use that is expensive or has a strong odour can be blended with other oils.

Any oil may cause an allergic reaction in certain people with highly sensitive skins. This very rarely happens but for safety's sake you could do a patch test first before making up your massage blend (see p. 57).

The following vegetable oils are among those used by aromatherapists:

ALMOND (SWEET) 🌿 My favourite. A light but nourishing oil suited to most skin types and soothing to any irritations. It contains vitamin E so keeps very well.

APRICOT KERNEL 🌿 Light texture, a good source of vitamins and minerals, but expensive and not easily obtainable.

ARACHIS 🌿 See Peanut.

AVOCADO 🌿 Heavy, rich in vitamins and readily absorbed. Specially good for dry or mature skins. It is best blended with a lighter oil.

COCONUT 🌿 The oil is fractionated, which means that during the pressing process it is heated and a fraction – the lighter oil – is extracted, leaving heavy fatty acids and wax behind. The resulting light-textured oil is becoming very popular, being non-greasy, easily absorbed and nourishing. Suitable for all skin types.

CORN ❦ Light texture, nourishing (contains vitamins and minerals). Inexpensive and suitable for all skin types.

GRAPESEED ❦ Light texture, odourless, easily absorbed. For all skin types, especially oily ones.

HAZELNUT ❦ Light texture, good penetrative power, contains vitamins and minerals. For all skin types, especially oily ones.

JOJOBA ❦ Really fine textured, but best blended with a lighter oil. Good for facial blends and troubled skin, i.e. acne, eczema, psoriasis. Rich in vitamin E. Stays fresh for longer than most oils – add it to massage oils to extend their life.

OLIVE ❦ Sticky, not a good lubricant, and has a strong odour. But this oil has healing properties, e.g. it is good for dry or sore skin. Best when added to other oils. Readily available.

PEACH KERNEL ❦ Light texture, contains useful nutrients, expensive. It is sometimes sold mixed with apricot-kernel oil (both are getting scarce).

PEANUT ❦ Also known as arachis oil. Rich in vitamins and minerals. Suitable for use on its own. Eases rheumatism of the joints.

SAFFLOWER • Light texture, good penetrative power, quite a good source of minerals and vitamins, cheap and readily available. For all skin types.

SESAME 🌿 Heavy texture, best added to other oils. The toasted variety is unsuitable, having a strong odour. The unrefined oil is a good source of vitamin E. This oil is reputed to help skin ailments and rheumatism.

SOYA 🌿 Light textured, inexpensive, but unless of good quality quickly turns rancid. It is nourishing, quickly absorbed and suitable for all skin types.

SUNFLOWER 🌿 Light texture, a source of minerals and vitamins, inexpensive. For all skin types.

VITAMIN E 🌿 Improves dry and mature skins and helps heal scars. Blend with other oils.

WHEATGERM 🌿 Dark with a pronounced odour, heavy and sticky, not a good lubricant, and expensive. Some people are allergic to wheatgerm. On the positive side, the oil is a rich source of vitamin E (improves dry skin, is good for healing burns and helps prevent scar tissue). Vitamin E is an anti-oxidant – a few drops added to your massage oils will prolong their shelf life.

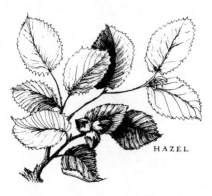

HAZEL

CHAPTER 5

Cautionary Notes

THIS IS a short chapter but a very important one. Before you use essential oils on yourself, your family or friends it is necessary to know when to exercise caution. But, provided you use common sense and take heed of the warnings given, essential oils are a very safe treatment for all kinds of conditions.

Special Cases

Babies and young children have delicate skin, so use the oils recommended as particularly gentle and suitable for them (see pp. 154 and 158).

During pregnancy, only certain oils are considered safe (see p. 144). Halve the amounts you would normally use. Avoid all others.

Epileptics or **anyone with brain damage** should not be given aniseed, star anise, camphor, fennel, hyssop, rosemary or sage.

There are oils that can be specially recommended for the elderly, see Chapter 13.

Asthmatics may be affected by certain essential oils; either consult a professional aromatherapist or use the recommended oils at low dosage.

Perhaps you have a **physically or mentally handicapped** child or older person to care for at home. If so, there is no reason why you should not give him/her aromatherapy treatment. At first, though, reduce the amount of essential oils in any given formula to about a half. You will soon get to know how he/she responds and can either increase or decrease amounts by a few drops if necessary.

Inhalation of essential oils can calm a troubled, perplexed mind, making it an ideal form of treatment for the handicapped. Consider arranging for the person to receive regular treatment from a professional aromatherapist. Nowadays therapists are using their skills with essential oils to improve communication and co-operation in areas that have proved difficult before. When the art of massage is used, words are not necessary; the caring touch is a better way of breaking down communication barriers.

Frequency of Use

I would advise taking a break from essential oils of at least 48 hours in any one week. But if you want to use them in the bath or in massage oils every day, drink extra water (this aids elimination of toxins). Restrict yourself to the mildest oils and reduce the recommended amounts by half.

Especially heed the cautions in Chapters 7 and 8 where you are exhorted to use certain oils in moderation – that means a maximum of 3–4 drops once or twice a week.

For therapy, it should not be necessary to use essential oils every day unless treating specific areas, such as painful joints or skin problems. As symptoms improve, the oils/lotions will be needed less often. Aromatherapy baths can be taken two or three times a week until the condition has significantly diminished, and then once or twice a week for maintenance.

Essence burners can be used on a daily basis because the oils are not in direct contact with the skin and are sufficiently diffused – it is still a good idea to drink extra water.

As a general rule, it is always wise to stop using essential oils for a while, and then to continue. I believe this helps stimulate the effect.

Toxicity and Side Effects

Certain citrus oils should not be used just prior to and during sunbathing because they are phototoxic. That means they may produce a change in skin pigmentation on exposure to ultra-violet light. Avoid using bergamot, lemon or lime when sunbathing. Other citrus oils – grapefruit, sweet orange, mandarin/tangerine – have been shown to have only a mild photosensitising effect though it would be as well to be cautious.

All spicy essential oils may irritate sensitive skins but are usually fine if used well diluted or in a blend.

Large doses of strong relaxing oils, in particular clary sage, can make some people feel drowsy. Remember this before using such oils on anyone who is soon after going to drive a car or use machinery.

Stop using any oil if an adverse reaction is felt.

Patch test

There is always the chance that a person may be allergic to any essential oil, even though it is one commonly regarded as safe. Anyone susceptible to allergy or who has a sensitive skin should test the oil in weak dilution on a small patch of skin before spreading it over a large area. If there is a skin reaction do not use it.

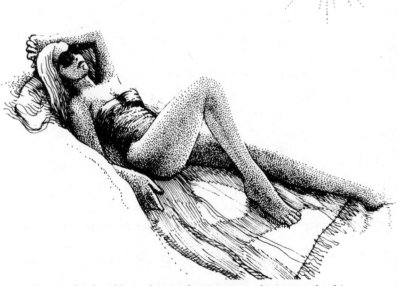

Citrus oils should not be used prior to or during sunbathing

Hazardous oils

Dangerously toxic essential oils are not normally available to the general public, but they are in existence and it is possible that a rogue company might sell them for use in aromatherapy. The list of potentially hazardous essential oils below has been compiled from general information on this subject. Those marked with an asterisk might be used by a professional aromatherapist who knows what she/he is doing. None of the oils on the list should be used by unqualified people as they could have serious side effects. *This warning applies to the essential oil, and not necessarily to the herb as used in cooking, herbal medicine or homoeopathic remedies.*

Arnica	*Arnica montana*
Bitter almond	*Prunus dulcis var. amara*
Boldo leaf	*Peumus boldus*
Broom	*Cytisus scoparius*
Buchu	*Barosma betulina*
Calamus	*Acorus calamus*
Cinnamon bark	*Cinnamomum cassia*
Camphor, brown and yellow	*Cinnamomum camphora*
*Camphor, white	" "
Chervil	*Anthriscus cerefolium*
Horseradish	*Cochlearia armoracia*
Jaborandi	*Pilocarpus microphyllus*
Melilotus	*Melilotus officinalis*
Mugwort	*Artemisia vulgaris*
Narcissus	*Narcissus poeticus*
Mountain (dwarf) pine	*Pinus mugo (P. pumilio)*
*Pennyroyal	*Mentha pulegium*
Rue	*Ruta graveolens*

Sassafras	*Sassafras variifolium*
Savine	*Juniperus sabina*
Tansy	*Tanacetum vulgare*
Thuja	*Thuja occidentalis*
Tonka	*Diperyx odorata oppositiflora*
Wintergreen	*Gaultheria procumbens*
Wormwood	*Artemisia absinthium*
Wormseed	*Chenopodium ambrosioides*

As the above essential oils are considered hazardous, you may well be asking why they are extracted at all, or listed in books. Many of them are indeed used in perfumes, food flavourings, medicines and medicinal products, but one hopes and assumes that they are harmless in these forms.

There is such a wide choice of essential oils that are safe to use at home that there is no reason to try to find or use any essential oil from the above list.

CHAPTER 6

Methods of Use

THE QUANTITIES OF OILS specified for the basic preparations in this chapter are just a guide. If you want to make up less, simply reduce proportionally the amount of carrier (base) oil and essential oils given in the formula, and of course proportionally more if you want to make up a larger quantity. The quantities given are for adults (see Chapters 11 and 12 for quantities to use in pregnancy and for children respectively).

Bear in mind that essential oils deteriorate when they are stored, and you must use suitable bottles to keep them in (see p. 43). If making a small quantity, say about an eggcupful, you can store it for a couple of days by covering with cling-film. For home use, you will probably not need to make up more than 100 ml of massage oil at a time, which is enough for three or four whole-body applications.

Conveniently, 1 tablespoon is approximately 25 ml, which is the amount of base oil needed for a full body massage for a person of average size. If you wish to apply a body oil after a bath or shower you will probably need less than 25 ml, unless you have a dry skin condition.

A 10 ml dropper bottle is convenient for measuring out drops of essential oils.

Massage Oils

Quantities: To 50 ml base oil, e.g. almond (*or* 35 ml almond + 15 ml wheatgerm, sesame or vitamin E oils) add 15–20 drops essential oil (a few extra won't hurt). You can use just one essential oil or several, but restrict your formula to four at the most.

Example: 10 drops lavender, 5 drops sandalwood, 5 drops ylang ylang. This is a good combination for a general purpose, after-bath-or-shower oil. It is relaxing as well as nourishing to the skin. (Use the same quantities if your base is a bland lotion or cream.)

NB: If you wish to use essential oils every day, choose the mildest ones and also reduce the recommended amounts by half.

Face Oils

Blend 20 ml at any one time, an amount that should last about one month. Apply face oil three times per week for general skin care, but if you are treating a specific skin complaint use it every night for two or three weeks, then reduce application to three times per week. If you do not like the feel of oil on your face, use a bland lotion or moisturising base.

I find using oil in the mornings very beneficial. This is one of my routines. I wash my face with a very rich honey soap, then I rinse and splash 10–15 times with warm water, pat dry with a towel and immediately apply face oil. By the time I am ready to apply make-up after, say, 20 minutes, the oil has penetrated. I thoroughly blot-dry any surface residue and apply a very light matt foundation. Using this method, I have found my make-up looks better and stays on longer.

My favourite face oil is a blend of sandalwood, neroli and lemon. I change the combinations occasionally because the skin gets used to the same treatment and needs a boost from time to time.

Guide to essential oils for different skin types	
Type of skin	*Essential oils*
Normal	Cedarwood, geranium, lavender, neroli, patchouli, sandalwood
Dry	Camomile, clary sage, geranium, jasmine, sandalwood, ylang ylang
Oily	Bergamot, eucalyptus, juniper, lavender, lemon, lemongrass (in very small doses, test for sensitivity), orange, peppermint, pine, rosemary
Sensitive	Camomile, jasmine, lavender, rose
Combination	Cedarwood, clary sage, lavender, ylang ylang
Mature	Clary sage, frankincense, myrrh, neroli
Wrinkled	Frankincense, lemon, neroli

Quantities: To 20 ml base oil, e.g. almond, or a blend of almond, jojoba and vitamin E, add 10 to 12 drops of essential oil. For oily skins, try a light coconut oil or grapeseed as the base.

Example: 4 drops lemon, 4 drops neroli, 4 drops sandalwood (anti-wrinkle formula for mature skins).

In the Bathroom

Using essential oils in the bath is a pleasurable way of doing oneself good. Essences do not dissolve in water, but that presents no real problem. One can agitate the water vigorously and persistently to disperse the oil as tiny globules. A better way is to take advantage of the oils' solubility in fats. There is fat of course in full cream milk, and after experimenting with different mediums I reckon milk is the best for dissolving essential oils. Add one cup of fresh milk to the water and swish it round. Then add your essential oils, give the water another good swish and imagine you are Cleopatra having your daily bath in asses' milk.

For convenience, you could keep a tin of powdered milk in the bathroom, though not ordinary skimmed milk powder. Full-cream powdered milk is not readily available but there is a skimmed milk on the market containing added vegetable fat which is perfectly suitable (it's what I use). Just half a cup of this in the bath water is sufficient.

For anyone who dislikes the idea of milk in their bath water, an alternative is to put in a tablespoon of a fine textured vegetable oil, such as almond or grapeseed, and then agitate well.

Do not add essences to hot running water – they will evaporate too quickly. Add them to the water just before you get in, but give it another good swish first.

To gain *maximum* benefit, wash first or take a quick shower. Then add your oils to clean bath water and just soak for 20 minutes in your wonderfully scented milk.

For specific treatments, such as for arthritis, stress, depression, skin problems, fatigue, and so on, the soaking method is by far the most effective – the introduction of soap to the skin will hinder the absorption of oils. For general use you can add essences to a bubble bath or bath salts.

With a strong sedative oil such as clary sage, it is best to have your bath at a time when you can relax totally afterwards – preferably at night before going to sleep. Four drops should be enough, unless you want to sleep for a week! (It is not advisable to go out immediately after an aromatherapy bath.)

Quantities guide: For adults in normal health, 6–8 drops; robust and healthy, up to 10 drops; frail adults or of weak constitution, 3–4 drops. For a baby's bath there are special instructions (see p. 154).

After-bath rest periods

Relaxation bath • 1½ hours.

Stimulating bath • have water cool – 20 minutes.

Arthritis/aches and pains/muscular problems • 1 hour.

Depression • 45 minutes–1 hour.

Fatigue, mental or physical • 1–2 hours.

General • 30 minutes.

Aphrodisiac • for two – as long as you like!

Essential oils are extra fast in effect when used in the bath because of absorption through the pores of the skin and by steam inhalation.

Aromatherapy shower

Some people have only a shower in their homes, not a bath, which makes life difficult where essential oils are concerned. Here are two methods you could use –

1   Put a flannel over the water outlet and sprinkle about 8 drops of essential oil over the shower base. As the steam rises you will inhale the oils.

2   Sprinkle about two or three drops of essence onto a warm, wet flannel and rub briskly over your body (avoiding sensitive areas).

If you only have a shower at your disposal, you should make more use of body oils.

Gargle

To make your own antiseptic gargle, to a cup of warm water add a teaspoonful of honey or salt and one drop of each of the following oils: geranium, lemon, tea-tree, thyme. Stir well to disperse the oils. (If more convenient, you could use 4 drops of just one of the oils suggested.)

Mouthwash

You can make an excellent mouthwash that not only freshens your mouth but is antiseptic and prevents bad breath (heavy smokers need this). See pp. 198–99.

Hair-oil conditioner

This is easily made by adding to a 20 ml bottle of almond, coconut or jojoba oil 10 drops of bay, 5 drops lavender and 5 drops rosemary. Stand the bottle in a container of hot water for two or three minutes (test oil for temperature before application). Massage into the hair and scalp, cover your hair with a plastic bag, then a towel, and leave for at least 20 minutes. Finally shampoo thoroughly, rinsing well.

Bidet

For any vaginal or genital irritations, or for haemorrhoids, add 4–6 drops of essential oils in your bidet or maybe a bowl suitable to sit on. It might prove uncomfortable to sit on either for more than five minutes. If this is the case, repeat the treatment three or four times a day. It is not necessary to dissolve the essences in milk or almond oil, unless you experience irritation.

Compresses

Hot compresses

These are very helpful when an area cannot be treated with oils, lotions or bathing owing to severe inflammation or weeping wounds. They are also very suitable for frail, elderly people. When massage is not advisable, conditions that can be treated with a compress include lumbago (if very painful), slipped disc (should not be massaged), painful, swollen joints, abscesses and boils, earache, period pains, diarrhoea, chest infections (especially in young babies and the elderly).

Large flannels, soft guest towels or lint can be used. The essential oils do not need to be dispersed by agitation of the water as it is necessary for the compress to pick up as much of the essence as possible. The water should be slightly hotter than bath water. Soak the compress, squeezing out excess water. Put the compress on the affected area and keep it in place with perhaps a plastic bag or tinfoil. After the compress has cooled it should be replaced by a fresh hot one.

Quantities: To 2 pints hot water add 10 to 15 drops of oil according to the specific condition. (For sensitive skins use only 6 to 8 drops; and young children 4 drops; babies, 1 to 2 drops.)

Cold compresses

Use exactly as in the method above except that the water should be cold from the refrigerator, and the compress can be kept in place with a bandage or plastic bag.

Cold compresses are useful for very inflamed conditions such as swollen arthritic joints, sprains, bruises, stings and bites, inflamed itchy skin, sunburn, headaches, hangovers and jet lag.

Hot and cold compresses

This is an ideal method to relieve sports injuries, especially sprained ankles. If this happens in your household (bloodless injuries), apply neat cajuput or tea-tree. Then apply as an instant cold compress a small packet of frozen peas from your freezer. Shake the peas so that they are loose, mould the packet to the injury and keep in place while you are preparing the hot and cold compresses.

When the cold compress is prepared, place it over the injury or inflammation. As the compress begins to lose its chill, replace with a hot compress. Do this about 7–8 times, ending with a cold compress that can be left in place. If the injury shows no sign of improving, seek medical advice.

If the particular condition is not acute, use compresses over a period of days.

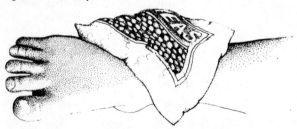

Inhalation

The old–fashioned method, and by far the best, is to use a basin, hot water, essences and a large towel. It is excellent for any breathing difficulties, chest infections, catarrh, sinusitis or headaches.

Pour a pint or two of near boiling water into a glass or china basin, let the steam subside a little and test it by putting your face over the steam about 10 or 12 inches away. When comfortable, add 4 or 5 drops of essential oil in the water and immediately put the towel over your head and basin leaving no air holes, keep your eyes closed and breath in the steam.

You will have to keep coming out for air and to blow your nose. If your eyes are sensitive, use sun-bed goggles or eye patches. This method of inhalation can sometimes take your breath away to begin with. Gradually build up inhalation time, i.e. inhale for 30 seconds, lift the towel, repeat for another 30 seconds, and so on until you have had a total of about 5 minutes. If possible, inhale for a further full 5 minutes.

Carefully supervise anyone with a very nervous disposition or who suffers with asthma, and also very young children and the very elderly. If you have broken capillaries (thread veins) on your face, do not use this method too often or for more than 2 minutes at any one time.

Essence Burners

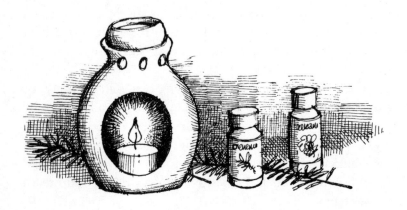

Essence burner

This is the most versatile and effective method of using essential oils and is authentic to the word AROMA THERAPY. Vaporising is considered by some to be the *only* method and other uses less effective. Inhalation of aromatic vapour certainly introduces the essential oils more quickly into the blood circulation than ingestion and, in some cases, external application. The diffusion of essences is greater and this is therefore considered a safer method of use.

The method of so-called 'burning' essential oils must be carried out correctly. The oils must be in water on a source of heat. As the oil vaporises its molecules are distributed around us and we inhale the aromatic, moisturised air.

The majority of essence burners have shallow dishes suggesting that the essential oil should be dropped neatly onto the heated pottery or metal. This, in my opinion, is inappropriate for therapy. The overall effect will be aromatic to a degree, but not as therapeutic or long-lasting as when the essential oils are heated in water. Too much heat denatures the oils.

The source of heat is generally a night-light candle in a metal container; it is placed in the main body of the burner with enough oxygen circulating to keep the flame at a balanced heat. Good quality night-lights last for about eight hours. The top container should hold just enough water to stay at the right temperature and usually evaporates after approximately two hours. It is advisable not to let the burner run dry; top it up with warm water (to avoid cracking), adding an extra drop or two of oil if necessary.

Some of the really expensive oils (jasmine, neroli, rose) are sold pre-blended with a vegetable oil such as jojoba; these are unsuitable for use in an essence burner.

For specific problems and ailments, blend the recommended oils in a bottle first, then add 6–10 drops of the mixture to a little water in the top container. Pre-formulated oils are readily available, saving time and effort.

Use your essence burner for conditions such as depression, tension, anxiety, poor memory, lack of concentration and brain fag. Physical ailments that respond well are headaches, sinusitis, catarrh, respiratory infections (colds, influenza, etc.).

Vaporised essential oils make delightful air fresheners and are completely ozone-friendly. You can create your own personal atmosphere, choosing perhaps clean, fresh, sparkling aromas or even seductive, sexy ones. If you need to put some spice back into your love life, tent the bedroom ceiling with red satin, get some eastern music, dress in a harem costume and blend coriander, sandalwood and ylang ylang in your essence burner. Conversely, if you need to tone down your loving activities, go to bed in curlers, bed socks and enough oil on your face to make you really slippery!

Once you realise the enormous benefits of using an essence burner you will want one in every room. Remember to put it somewhere safe, especially if there are children in the house.

Vaporising ring

An alternative means of burning essential oils is the vaporising ring. Widely available from health stores and other outlets, you may have wondered how it is used.

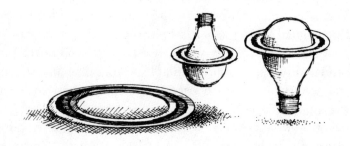

Vaporising ring

Place the ring on a flat surface, put a few drops of perfume oil into the groove. When the ring has absorbed the oil, place it on a light-bulb (60 watt max.) and switch on the light.

The ring may be used on either a table lamp or on a

pendant light. In the case of the latter, unscrew the bulb, slip the ring over it and re-screw the bulb into the socket.

This method of vaporising is not as effective as an essence burner for the relief of symptoms, but it's fine if you simply want to create a nice aroma in a room.

Neat Essential Oils

There are a few instances where essences can be used without preparation.

A few drops of neat lavender oil on your pillow is an effective way to relieve insomnia. Put two or three drops of the oil on either side and in the middle of the pillow, so that when you turn over in the night you'll still get a whiff. Make sure you do not get the oil into your eyes as this will irritate; it should be about 6 inches from your nose. Ylang ylang, camomile, marjoram or sandalwood can be used in the same way as lavender. They will not stain (unless adulterated or synthetic).

If you are suffering from a headache or nasal catarrh and you have no access to a burner, put a drop or two of essence on a handkerchief or cotton-wool pad and continually waft it under your nose. Alternatively, put a few drops of essence on your shirt – if it is not an expensive one – about 6 inches from your chin.

In an emergency situation, essential oils can be used like smelling salts – pass the bottle just beneath the nose. This procedure can also be used in severe cases of nasal congestion.

Tea-tree oil can be applied neat to athlete's foot and fungal infections of the nails three times a day for about one week until symptoms are relieved.

Dab unsightly pustules, boils and spots with tea-tree or lavender oil on a cotton-wool bud.

Essential oils are a great help in first aid. Some can be used neat for a short time (see p. 193).

For Use Around the House

Essential oils can be used either on their own or in conjunction with proprietary household products. Oils of pine, lemon, lavender, orange, tea-tree or thyme can be used as disinfectants. Add them to hot water for a general wipe-over disinfectant, or to floor-washing/rinsing water. A few drops of lemon, lavender, orange or pine can be dropped into your sink drainage. I always sprinkle a few drops of pine or lavender into the loo.

When washing clothes, essences can be added to the rinsing water (three or four drops to an average sized bowl). A few drops can also be added to your fabric conditioner in the washing machine.

It is a good idea to drop a little pine or lemon on the clothes or bedding of someone who is ill in the family.

The oils I have mentioned for household use are not expensive, and if you buy large quantities (50 or 100 ml) you will find that most suppliers will give you a discount.

You can easily make your own flower water using essential oils. Genuine flower waters come from the distillation process (rose, lavender, orange-flower), but these are not always available and can be expensive. You will need a large glass bottle (about 200 ml), preferably amber. Use pure spring water and 3–4 drops of your favourite oil. Choose, for example, from camomile, geranium, jasmine, lavender, lemon, mandarin, neroli, orange (sweet), rose and ylang ylang. Shake the bottle vigorously and keep it in a cool, dark place. Continue to shake it well two or three times a day or every time you pass it. In approximately 10 days you will have a lightly perfumed flower water which can be used as a face rinse or spray. Lavender, camomile, rose, lemon or orange water can be used in the making of sweets such as fondants or icings.

For Animals

To bathe a wound or abscess, to half a pint of cooled boiled water add 3 drops lavender, or 4 drops tea-tree, or 3 drops lemon oil, or a desertspoon of pure squeezed lemon juice (not bottled juice). Incidentally, tea-tree is an important ingredient in a well-known veterinary skin balm.

To get rid of fleas, tea-tree oil should be rubbed on your hands and then rubbed through the fur of your dog or cat (they don't like the smell too much, but neither do the fleas!). Tea-tree oil is non-poisonous and will not hurt the animal when it grooms itself. Fleas do not like the smell of garlic, either. If you can obtain oil of garlic rub it through the fur and the fleas will stay away, but the cat will find it difficult to find a willing lap.

Oil of citronella sprinkled around your garden plants is reputed to stop pussy digging. Hiding strips of paper impregnated with citronella may stop determined claws being exercised on your carpets or chairs (you will have to impregnate the strips regularly as the aroma wears off). You can buy scratching posts for your beloved moggy impregnated with cat mint, which all cats adore. The idea is that, attracted to the smell, the cat obligingly sharpens its claws on the post and not on your furniture. But my ginger Tom slobbers, cuddles, sits and sleeps on his catmint post and wouldn't dream of scratching it – only Victorian armchairs are good enough for that.

CHAPTER 7

Getting to Know Essential Oils

BECAUSE THERE ARE SO MANY essential oils on the market, it is difficult to know where to start and end. This chapter deals, in some detail, with 25 of the more popular and well-known essential oils, which have also proved to be invaluable in my aromatherapy practice. In my opinion, they are all suitable for home use provided all instructions are followed. They present a varied and useful selection and are widely available. However, if you have difficulty in obtaining any of them, details of some reputable suppliers are given on p. 223.

Before using any essential oils it is very important to read the cautions given in Chapter 5 and listed against individual oils. This will prevent unnecessary problems, such as skin irritation or minor side effects.

BERGAMOT ❀ *(Citrus bergamia)*

An olive-green oil obtained by expression or steam distillation from the peel of a citrus fruit native to Calabria in southern Italy. The plant is a small tree and should not be confused with the herbaceous plant of the same name, which is also called bee balm (*Monarda* species). Its lively fresh aroma is quite distinctive – it is the scent in Earl Grey tea, and is also used in eau de Cologne.

Methods of use • Bath, essence burner, massage oil (test skin for sensitivity).

Caution • This oil is phototoxic, so do not use it whilst sunbathing or before exposing yourself to the sun. Do not use the oil if there are raised moles on the skin. Bergamot can irritate sensitive skins. For regular skin application, use Bergamot F.C.F. (i.e. fourocoumarin free).

Healing effects • (Action: antispasmodic, antidepressant, deodorant, expectorant, nerve tonic.)

Uplifting, calming and relaxing without a sedative effect. Gives a sensation of slow motion, rather like floating. Promotes a feeling of love and peace. I find it helps with problems of indecision, as well as bringing harmony and balance to the psyche (inner mind/soul). It relieves tension, anxiety, extreme negativity, depression. Use it especially when there is a need to release emotional problems.

In massage oils or lotions, bergamot can heal skin problems, such as eczema, psoriasis, acne and oily conditions. For this purpose it is best mixed with other oils (see recipe sections).

For sore throats and bad breath, bergamot can be used in a gargle or mouthwash respectively (do not swallow).

Treat bronchitis with chest rubs or inhalation.

It is thought that bergamot regulates thyroid gland activity.

Bergamot is considered safe to use throughout pregnancy.

CAJUPUT ❧ *(Melaleuca leucadendron, M. minor)*

This colourless or very pale yellow oil comes from the leaves and twigs of a medium sized tree native to India. It has a powerful, fresh, herbaceous scent with eucalyptus tones.

Methods of use • Bath, compress, essence burner, massage oil.

Caution • Can cause slight irritation to sensitive skins.

Healing effects • (Action: analgesic, antiseptic, rubefacient, stimulant.)

Cajuput is one of the best natural analgesics. It blends and works well with other oils and can also be used successfully on its own. For toothache, add 5–6 drops of cajuput to a warm compress and apply to the face around the affected area. This will dull the pain. For sprains and bruises, apply a little neat oil as first aid only. In the long term, treat with diluted oil either in compresses or lotions.

The oil has a mild diuretic effect on injuries that are prone to fluid build-up.

Use cajuput diluted in almond oil to soothe sunburn.

Other physical conditions that often respond to cajuput include: acne, arthritis, asthma, bronchitis, dental neuralgia, dermatitis, earache, eczema, gout, headaches, laryngitis, period pains, psoriasis, rheumatism, sore throats, torn ligaments.

Mentally, cajuput has a stimulating, invigorating effect. And I find this oil works well on emotions when dealing with a painful experience, whether recent or not.

In pregnancy, cajuput may be considered safe to use after four months.

CAMOMILE, TRUE (ROMAN) ❦
(Chamaemelum nobile, formerly Anthemis nobilis)
CAMOMILE, WILD (GERMAN) ❦ *(Matricaria recutita, formerly M. chamomilla, Chamomilla recutita)*

These two species of camomile are widely used in aromatherapy and their properties are very similar. The oil is extracted by steam distillation from the flowers of German camomile and from the whole plant of Roman camomile. The oil of the former species is deep blue and the aroma is sweet herbaceous, like strong honey, with fruity undertones. The oil of the latter is paler and a greener blue, the aroma being sweet herbaceous, and like tea. The blue colour of camomile oil turns green with age.

Methods of use • Bath, compress, essence burner, massage oil or lotion.

Caution • A mild emmenagogue; in pregnancy, avoid during first seven months.

Healing effects • (Action: antiseptic, anti-inflammatory, astringent, antispasmodic, diuretic, emmenagogue, febrifuge, hepatic, sedative.)

The healing effect of camomile on the skin is due to a blue substance called azulene that it contains (especially the German camomile). It eases inflammation, eruptions or ulceration, e.g. acne, burns, eczema and psoriasis.

The herb was used in folk medicine to reduce fevers. In aromatherapy it is effective in treating the following physical conditions: arthritis and rheumatism, digestive problems, liver congestion, muscular cramps and spasm. It may also be used for period irregularities, PMT and menopausal problems.

It has a soothing and calming effect both on irritable children and grumpy adults. Anger, rage, anguish, severe tension and obsessiveness are negative emotions that may be alleviated by this oil.

CEDARWOOD

CEDAR, ATLAS 🌺 *(Cedrus atlantica)*
CEDAR, RED (VIRGINIA) 🌺 *(Juniper virginiana)*

The oil of more than one type of tree is sold as cedarwood. The Atlas cedar is a true cedar and closely related to the cedar of Lebanon *(Cedrus libani),* which unfortunately no longer grows in abundance (only a few hundred survive). The oil from the wood is pale yellow. It has a soft, warm woody fragrance, with sandalwood undertones that are sweeter and stronger.

Red (Virginian) cedarwood oil is recognised by its very woody aroma reminiscent of pencils.

Method of use • Bath, essence burner, massage oil or lotion.

Caution • Cedarwood oil is abortive and should not be used during pregnancy.

Healing effects • (Action: antiseptic, astringent, diuretic, expectorant, sedative.)

Oil of cedarwood, as an astringent, is good for acne and oily skin conditions, eczema and psoriasis. Mixed with lemon oil it helps relieve sinusitis and breathing difficulties such as catarrh and bronchitis. It is a remedy for urinary infections, and is also useful as a stimulant in cases of low sexual response due to nervous tension.

Cedarwood uplifts the spirit and aids meditation. The mental effect is sedative, harmonising, strengthening and soothing. If you suffer from low self-esteem or lack confidence, cedarwood may help.

Personally, I find Atlas cedarwood superior in effect.

CLARY SAGE ❧ *(Salvia sclarea)*

The plant is in the same family as the common sage *(Salvia officinalis)*, the oil of which is considered toxic and is not recommended for general use. Clary sage, however, is comparatively free from toxicity. Obtained from the flowering tops, it is pale yellow with a herbaceous, hay-like aroma, warm, musky and strong.

Methods of use • Bath, essence burner, massage oil or lotion.

Caution • Use in moderation. Large amounts can cause drowsiness. In pregnancy, avoid until after seven months.

Healing effects • (Action: antiseptic, antispasmodic, astringent, emmenagogue, sedative, antidepressant.)

Clary sage is renowned for its sedative effect. The drowsiness it might cause can last for several days. However, after it has had time to reduce anxiety, it becomes restorative to the whole system, recharging the emotional and physical batteries. Use less clary sage than other oils because it is very strong.

A clary sage bath before going to bed will help dissolve any stress and muscular tension.

Clary sage is helpful in PMT and menopause problems. To ease period pains, mix clary sage with cajuput and camomile in a massage oil or lotion and apply to the abdomen. Alternatively, use the same essential oils in a warm compress.

During labour, use a clary sage compress on the abdomen, and a few drops in the burner.

I find clary sage benefits mature skins.

For troubled sleep, massage the solar plexus area (middle diaphragm, just below the ribs) and the feet with diluted clary sage and lavender.

Clary sage is wonderful at times of extreme anguish, depression, panic or shock; it will help you see your problems in perspective. Use it for mental and physical debility.

CYPRESS, ITALIAN ❦ *(Cupressus sempervirens)*

This cypress is native to the Mediterranean region. The pale yellow, almost colourless oil is distilled from the needles, twigs and cones. Its refreshing aroma, similar to pine, is a little spicy with woody tones.

Methods of use • Bath, bidet, footbath, essence burner, massage oil or lotion.

Healing effects • (Action: antiseptic, antispasmodic, astringent, deodorant, diuretic, nerve tonic.)

Cypress has been used in medicine for thousands of years and was thought to be a remedy used by Hippocrates (the father of medicine). The oil has a warming, balancing effect on the body systems and is relaxing without causing drowsiness. It has a refreshing, uplifting and regenerating effect, calming irritability and impatience. Cypress can sometimes help with indecision.

The oil has an astringent effect on haemorrhoids and varicose veins. It alleviates menstrual and menopausal problems. For hot flushes, before going to bed, try a foot massage with equal parts of cypress and clary sage diluted in almond oil.

Use cypress as a skin tonic for an oily skin, and in a footbath when there is an odour problem.

In pregnancy, cypress may be considered safe to use after four months.

EUCALYPTUS ❀ *(Eucalyptus globulus)*

The hundreds of species of eucalyptus are mostly native to Australia. They range in height from small shrubs under 10 feet to the tallest known broad-leafed tree *(E. regnans)* reaching nearly 400 feet. The oil used in aromatherapy comes from *E. globulus*, otherwise known as the southern blue gum, which can grow to over 100 feet tall. Almost colourless, this oil which comes from the leaves and twigs has a very powerful, readily recognisable smell with a camphoraceous note.

Methods of use • Bath, essence burner, inhalant, massage oil.

Healing effects • (Action: analgesic, antiseptic, antispasmodic, deodorant, diuretic, expectorant, mental stimulant, rubefacient.)

Eucalyptus is an age-old remedy for colds and flu, due to its decongestant, anti-viral and bactericidal action. It is also helpful in urinary tract infections, asthma, rheumatism and for muscular aches and pains.

The psychological effect of eucalyptus can be summed up as stimulating and uplifting. If you are feeling lethargic or low in spirits, eucalyptus may be just what you need.

Eucalyptus is an effective insect repellant.

In pregnancy, eucalyptus may be considered safe to use after 4 months.

FENNEL, SWEET ❀ *(Foeniculum vulgare)*

The oil from this herb native to the Mediterranean region is extracted from the seeds by steam distillation. Very pale yellow in colour, its aroma is sweet, delicate but penetrating, and reminiscent of aniseed.

Methods of use • Bath, essence burner, massage oil.

Caution • Use in moderation. Large doses over a long period could produce side effects. The oil should not be used on very young children or on sensitive skin. It should not be used by people with epilepsy. Avoid it during pregnancy.

Healing effects • (Action: antiseptic, antispasmodic, carminative, emmenagogue, expectorant, digestive, diuretic, stimulant.)

Fennel has been used in medicine for thousands of years and was believed to impart strength and fortitude. Eating the seed helped dispel flatulence. It was also supposed to reduce obesity and promote the flow of milk in nursing mothers. Its hormonal effect is used to relieve menopause and menstrual problems. Use a few drops of fennel in almond oil as a soothing massage oil for the abdomen.

Fennel oil used either in the bath or as a massage rub reduces excess fluid caused by hormonal imbalances (fennel tea should be drunk as well). It is valuable in the treatment of cellulitis.

Fennel may be used in cases of weakness of character, insecurity, fear, worry and moodiness.

FRANKINCENSE ❀ *(Boswellia thurifera)*

Also known as olibanum, or sometimes gum thus, it is extracted by steam distillation from the resin of a small African tree. The oil is amber or greeny-yellow in colour with a warm, spicy, slightly peppery scent.

Methods of use • Bath, compress, essence burner, lotion or massage oil.

Healing effects • (Action: antiseptic, astringent, cicatrising, diuretic, sedative, tonic.)

Frankincense is exceptional for skin care, revitalising and rejuvenating the tissues, giving a healthy glow and keeping wrinkles at bay. For excessive menstrual bleeding, I recommend using frankincense in a compress, or diluted in an almond oil base and gently applied to the abdomen.

Thousands of years ago, frankincense was used in rituals for purification and the exorcism of evil spirits. I believe that Frankincense has the same effect on our body and mind, cleansing negative thoughts – fear, resentment, worry and confusion – replacing them with a feeling of well-being and tranquillity.

In pregnancy, frankincense may be considered safe to use after four months.

GERANIUM ❀ *(Pelargonium odorantissimum, P. graveolens, P. capitatum* and other species)

This essential oil is derived from the type of geranium grown in garden tubs and window-boxes, more correctly named pelargoniums, and very widely cultivated. Obtained by steam distillation, the oil is a pale soft green with a sweet floral scent that varies depending on the species used.

Methods of use • Bath, essence burner, lotion, massage oil.

Caution • May irritate very sensitive skins.

Healing effects • (Action: antidepressant, antiseptic, astringent, circulatory stimulant, diuretic, hypotensive, sedative, tonic.)

Geranium oil stimulates the adrenal glands, promoting natural balance of hormones, which is a great help for menopause troubles and pre-menstrual tension.

The oil is particularly useful in many types of skin conditions: burns, ulcers, wounds, dermatitis, eczema, psoriasis and inflammation.

The effect of geranium oil on the mind is calming and uplifting. It strengthens the personality by increasing confidence and self-esteem.

The oil combats mood swings, tension, tearfulness and depression.

In pregnancy, geranium may be considered safe to use after four months

GRAPEFRUIT 🌿 *(Citrus paradisi)*

Essential oil of grapefruit, obtained from the peel, is becoming increasingly popular among aromatherapists. It mainly comes from the USA and has a fresh, bright, tangy aroma just like the fruit.

Methods of use: Bath, essence burner, massage oil or lotion.

Caution • Can irritate sensitive skins and is mildly phototoxic.

Healing effects • (Action: diuretic, lymphatic stimulant, general stimulant, tonic.)

Grapefruit uplifts mind, body and spirit. It combats both physical and mental tiredness – jet lag in particular – restoring energy levels. It feels very cooling in hot weather. You will find it helpful in common ailments such as fluid retention due to overweight, PMT and menopause problems. It also stimulates the lymphatic system and helps eliminate toxins. Use it to ease anxiety and lift depression; it can clear confusion and indecision, and sharpens the mind.

The oil is also useful for freshening rooms, especially after smokers have been in them. It reduces animal odours and cooking smells.

Grapefruit may be considered safe to use throughout pregnancy.

JASMINE 🌿 *(Jasminum officinale, J. grandiflorum)*

Jasmine absolute is extremely expensive. Large quantities of flowers are needed to produce a small amount of oil. However, its exquisite aroma – sweet, floral, with almost

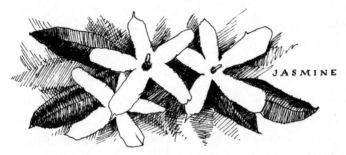

JASMINE

harsh honey-like tones – is so strong that very little is needed. It is dark brown in colour.

Methods of use • Bath, face oil, lotion. If you feel extravagant, it can be used in an essence burner. However, the oil is mostly sold in jojoba base which is not suitable for burning.

Healing effects • (Action: antidepressant, antiseptic, antispasmodic, sedative.)

Like rose oil, jasmine has a wonderful effect on the skin regardless of type or age. Jasmine relaxes muscles that are stiff and tight from anxiety and tension. It is wonderfully relaxing when used in the bath. Often people who suffer from extreme anguish are so-called chilly mortals; this chilliness is caused by blocked energy. Jasmine is of great help in warming the spirit and releasing blockage. Regular use of jasmine helps raise self-esteem, increases confidence and imparts a feeling of well-being.

Jasmine is believed to stimulate creativity and original ideas! Used at night it induces sleep and brings forth wonderful dreams.

In pregnancy, jasmine may be considered safe to use after four months. During labour, use in a compress across the lower abdomen.

LAVENDER 🌸 *(Lavandula angustifolia, also known as L. officinalis and L. spica)*

See also Lavandin (p. 113).

The common or old English lavender originated in the Mediterranean region but is grown commercially in several countries, including England and France. Its delightful aroma is familiar to everyone. The oil, colourless or pale yellow, is obtained by steam distillation and could be described as herbaceous and floral with woody undertones.

Methods of use • Bath, compresses, essence burner, lotion, massage oil. It can also be used neat as first aid. A drop or two on the pillow will aid restful sleep.

Caution • A mild emmenagogue; in pregnancy, avoid for the first seven months.

Healing effects • (Action: analgesic, antispasmodic, antiseptic, cicatrising, deodorant, diuretic, emmenagogue, expectorant, hypotensive, sedative.)

A favourite aromatic for thousands of years, there certainly does not appear to be many conditions lavender cannot help. Versatile and safe, it is ideal for home use. Keep a bottle handy for all kinds of emergency. In the event of a cut, burn, bite or sting, apply neat lavender oil directly on the affected part – it will rapidly relieve pain and heal the tissue. Lavender will act as a bacteriacidal agent for the treatment of acne. Apply neat oil to the spot with the tip of a cotton-wool bud. Although safe to use neat on a troubled area, lavender will dry the skin if over-used.

After many years of using lavender, I am still amazed at how many everyday problems good old lavender helps. It can soothe and calm all kinds of nervous tension and shock, helping to lift depression, dispel irritability, and quell panic and hysteria. A few drops rubbed on the forehead soothes a headache. Try it to alleviate muscular aches and pains, arthritic and rheumatic pain, cramp, dermatitis, eczema, dry skin, oily skin, sunburn, sinusitis, colds, influenza, bronchitis, asthma, high blood pressure, insomnia, mental debility and anxiety.

In pregnancy, lavender may be considered safe to use after seven months, and during labour.

LEMON ❧ *(Citrus limonum)*

The lemon tree, a native of South-east Asia, was introduced to Italy about some 1500 years ago, whence its cultivation has spread throughout the Mediterranean region and to other parts of the world. The greenish-yellow oil is expressed from the rind.

Methods of use • Bath, essence burner, massage oil or lotion. The juice of a lemon can be used neat as an antiseptic, or diluted in water as a gargle.

Caution • Citrus oils can cause skin irritations and are phototoxic (see p. 56).

Healing effects • (Action: antiseptic, astringent, mildly diuretic, expectorant, hepatic, hypotensive, mental stimulant, tonic.)

Lemon is a very important essential oil and, like lavender, it helps numerous conditions. Because of its antiseptic action, lemon oil is useful for treating respiratory tract infections – colds, sore throats, influenza, bronchitis and sinusitis. For tonsilitis, gargle with lemon juice in warm water. Bathe infected wounds with diluted lemon juice or oil. It can relieve heaches and migraine (try slices of lemon on the forehead).

Lemon stimulates the circulation and is therefore considered helpful in treating varicose veins.

Traditionally, lemon juice is squeezed over fish and shellfish, as it combats bacterial contamination. We are constantly being warned about the dangers of pathogenic bacteria in the foods that we buy, so I always cook poultry and fish with whole lemons, plenty of garlic and fresh rosemary.

Try oil of lemon to ease asthma, gingevitis (inflammation of the gums) and liverishness, and to help get rid of warts and verrucas, and vaginal thrush.

For skin care, essential oil of lemon added to almond oil or a bland cream acts as a cleanser, toner and a great anti-wrinkle agent. A drop of the oil added to toothpaste will keep your teeth sparkling white.

Lemon oil has a stabilising effect on the emotions and helps treat anxiety. Inhaling the vapour of lemon oil connects the spirit and the body to the higher self.

Lemon may be considered safe to use throughout pregnancy.

MARJORAM, SWEET ❧ *(Origanum marjorana)*

A pale yellowish, spicy oil is obtained from the flowering tops and leaves of this well-known European herb.

Methods of use • Bath, essence burner, massage oil or lotion, drops on pillow.

Caution • Over-use could cause a stupefying effect. Avoid during pregnancy.

Healing effects • (Action: analgesic, antispasmodic, antiseptic, emmenagogue, expectorant, sedative.)

Marjoram has a warming effect on the body which is effective on muscular spasm, arthritis and rheumatism. Mix it with lavender, camomile and cajuput, to make a soothing lotion to relieve the pain of all kinds of muscular problems, especially cramp.

The oil is often alleviates headaches and migraine, and calms the digestive system.

Marjoram has a soothing and fortifying effect on the mind and in times of grief can impart warmth and strength. It will also help feelings of loneliness and depression.

MELISSA (LEMON BALM) ❦ *(Melissa officinalis)*

Native to southern Europe though widely grown elsewhere, the lemon balm plant yields only minute quantities of oil. This makes it difficult to obtain and also extremely expensive to buy. World production can be as little as 2 kilograms. However, it is possible to purchase a therapeutically identical melissa oil reconstructed out of the natural plant components. This is considered to be a reconstructed oil, not a synthetic. It has a sharp, sweet, strong lemon aroma.

Sometimes melissa is cut with lemongrass or citronella. A synthetically produced melissa oil is supplied to the perfume industry – one hopes this type is never sold to aromatherapists. Lemon or lemon-grass is often mixed with the genuine oil to bring down the cost.

Methods of use • Bath, essence burner, massage oil or lotion.

Caution • Can irritate very sensitive skins.

Healing effects • (Action: antispasmodic, digestive, sedative, tonic.)

Uplifting, calming, soothing, the herb has been used for hundreds of years as an 'elixir of life'.

A heart tonic, melissa also relieves symptoms of anxiety, panic and shock. It clears the mind and raises the spirits. .

You can enjoy melissa as a herbal tea. Steep one ounce of the leaves in one pint of boiling water. Let the tea stand for 15–20 minutes. Add honey and either drink warm or chilled.

Melissa may be considered safe to use throughout pregnancy.

NEROLI (ORANGE BLOSSOM) ❦ *(Citrus aurantium)*

Neroli is distilled from the blossoms of the bitter orange tree. The colour of neroli oil is pale yellow and the aroma is clean floral in type with bitter-sweet undertones.

Methods of use • An essence burner would be ideal but unfortunately neroli is very expensive, so use it in the bath or in a massage or face oil. Neroli is often sold blended with an oil such as jojoba, but this is unsuitable for an essence burner.

Healing effects • (Antidepressant, antiseptic, antispasmodic, cicatrising, sedative.)

Neroli has a profound effect on the nervous system, calming muscle spasm, especially in the heart area. If the condition is due to tension, try neroli as a massage oil or lotion and rub the chest muscles. Do not attempt to treat a heart condition – seek medical advice.

The euphoric effect of neroli is similar to that of clary sage. It helps strengthen the nerves and is a general tonic. Used in a face oil at night, it will help induce peaceful sleep as well as rejuvenate the skin (especially mature, dry types).

Neroli helps balance mood swings. It can be used to combat a tendency to tearfulness, nervous tension, hypochondria and phobias, and also menopause and PMT troubles.

In pregnancy, neroli may be considered safe to use after four months.

PATCHOULI ❀ *(Pogostemon patchouli)*

Patchouli comes from the leaves of a bushy herb native to the Far East. It is a member of the Labiatae family (which includes nettles, mints, lavenders and sages). This oil is a dark brownish yellow, and the aroma can be described as balsamic, sweet woody and musty. It is a mysterious oil that some will find a little medicinal in aroma – you either love it or hate it. Blended with other oils, patchouli gives depth and body; it goes particularly well with ylang ylang and sweet orange.

Methods of use • Bath, compress, essence burner, massage oil.

Caution • None apparent.

Healing effects • (Antidepressant, diuretic, sedative.)

In the 'Swinging Sixties' patchouli was a very popular perfume; the message of 'flower power' was love and harmony, and this is exactly what the essential oil of patchouli imparts. It can stabilise and calm an anguished state, and is helpful at times of indecision and whenever dealing with major changes in life.

Excellent for skin care, especially for dry, cracked skin, the oil also makes a very soothing massage oil. It can also help reduce fluid retention.

In pregnancy, patchouli may be considered safe to use after four months.

PEPPERMINT ❧ *(Mentha piperata)*
The oil of peppermint is obtained by steam distillation from the whole herb. It contains menthol, hence its distinctive smell.

Methods of use • Bath, essence burner, massage oil or lotion.

Caution • Can induce disturbed sleep or nightmares if used in large amounts late at night.

Healing effects • (Action: analgesic, antiseptic, antispasmodic, expectorant, hepatic, mental stimulant, nerve tonic.)

Peppermint is well known for its effect on the digestive system, easing nausea, stomach cramps and diarrhoea. It also relieves period pain and headaches. As an exception to the general rule, the oil can be taken internally – but only a couple of drops, either on sugar or in a cup of warm water.

Peppermint is stimulating and uplifting, and can help with feelings of lethargy, increasing the impetus to get on with things. It can also help release deep fears and suppressed anger that would otherwise affect the liver and spleen.

Like lavender, peppermint is a must for the first aid cupboard as well as for the pleasure of its aroma.

In pregnancy, peppermint may be considered safe to use after four months.

PETITGRAIN ❦ *(Citrus aurantium)*

An oil obtained from the leaves and twigs of the bitter orange tree (neroli comes from the blossoms, see p. 94). Originally petitgrain was extracted from the still tiny unripe fruits, looking like 'little grains' – hence the name.

The aroma is fresh and green with a hint of neroli.

Methods of use • Bath, essence burner, massage oil or lotion, hair rinse.

Healing effects • A tonic for the nervous system, digestive system and skin, petitgrain is similar to neroli though less sedative, and less costly. It alleviates anxiety, nervous exhaustion and stress-related conditions, especially insomnia. Neroli, however, is to be preferred in serious or acute cases of anxiety.

Some aromatherapists have found that petitgrain helps patients reduce their dependence on tranquillisers.

This oil is a good remedy for flatulence and dyspepsia caused by a so-called 'nervous stomach'. It is also helpful in the treatment of acne and greasy skin conditions.

Petigrain often aids recovery from illness. On the mental and spiritual level, it lifts negative conditions, enabling positive energy to clear the mind of doubt and fear.

In pregnancy, petitgrain may be considered safe to use after four months.

ROSE ❧ *(Rosa damascena; R. centifolia)*

The oil from *Rosa damascena*, the damask rose, comes mainly from Bulgaria. Known as rose otto or attar of roses, the essential oil is now obtained by steam distillation.

The absolute (from solvent extraction) is obtained from the *Rosa centifolia*, notably cultivated in the Grasse area of France and also Morocco, for perfumery.

Pure Bulgarian rose oil is one of the most expensive oils used in aromatherapy (about £80 for 5 ml). But it is strong and only a drop or two needs to be used at a time, so it will last a long while. Rose absolute is a deep reddish brown in colour and thick in consistency (frequently solid at room temperature). Sometimes the essential oil of rose is a dilution of the absolute. Unfortunately, there are a lot of adulterations and synthetic copies on the market. When you smell true rose oil it penetrates your mind and you feel like soaring to the heights of heaven. Rosewater is obtained by distillation. A few reputable companies make a blend of true rose oil in jojoba, which preserves the delicate essential oil, and is ready to use at an affordable price.

Methods of use • Essence burner (if you are wealthy). A few drops in the bath is pure joy. For a face oil, buy rose oil blended in jojoba.

Caution • In pregnancy, avoid for the first seven months.

Healing effects • (Action: antidepressant, antiseptic, antispasmodic, cicatrising, circulatory stimulant, emmenagogue, hepatic, sedative and nerve tonic.)

Rose oil is healing for a great many conditions: circulation problems, broken capillaries, varicose veins, arthritis, rheumatism, hormone imbalances, PMT, menstrual and menopause problems.

Rose oil is excellent for skin care. All skin types benefit, especially the dry, sensitive sort. Skin ailments such as eczema, psoriasis and acne may be improved with rose oil. Pure rosewater is refreshing and soothing as a toner.

This oil also soothes fear, anxiety, feelings of anger, frustration and resentment, jealousy and suspicion. It lifts depression and helps to clarify the mind, leading to positive decisions. In short, it is a wonderful tonic for heart and soul.

ROSEMARY ❧ *(Rosmarinus officinalis)*

The rosemary plant is a small evergreen shrub with narrow, leathery, greyish green leaves and pale violet-blue flowers. It is a member of the Labiatae family, which includes the nettles and sages. A native of Mediterranean countries, rosemary has been used in herbal medicine for many centuries. The essential oil is distilled from the leaves and flowering tops. Its colour is pale yellow and its aroma is herbaceous, powerful, and like a mixture of lavender and camphor. Rubbing rosemary leaves between the fingers will readily release the aroma.

Rosemary oil is one of the traditional ingredients of eau de Cologne.

Methods of use • Bath, compress, essence burner, massage oil, steam inhalation.

Caution • Avoid during the first seven months of pregnancy. Rosemary should also be avoided by epileptics and by people suffering from high blood pressure.

Healing effects • (Action: analgesic, antiseptic, antispasmodic, astringent, circulatory stimulant, rubefacient, tonic.)

Essential oil of rosemary is marvellous to use the day before long, vigorous exercise, as it will help to prevent muscular strain. It has pain-relieving properties. Use it to ease muscular stiffness and aches, arthritis and gout, headaches and neuralgia. Skin problems such as acne, dermatitis and eczema respond well to rosemary. This oil tones the skin and is especially suitable for oily complexions.

Rosemary helps eliminate toxins trapped in the fatty tissues of the body and helps reduce water retention. It is valuable, too, for respiratory problems – colds, bronchitis, sinusitis, asthma – for which steam inhalation is recommended (see p. 69).

Rosemary has a stimulating effect on the blood vessels, helping a poor circulation, and is a well-known remedy for hair loss. It is also said to stimulate the brain! Certainly it is effective for mental fatigue and poor memory. William Shakespeare wrote: 'There's rosemary, that's for remembrance...' *(Hamlet).*

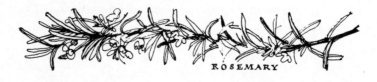

ROSEMARY

SANDALWOOD 🌻 *(Santalum album)*

Essential oil of sandalwood is obtained by steam distillation of chippings from the heartwood of a small tree native to India. It has been used from time immemorial as incense and in perfumes. The rich, sweet aroma has woody undertones. It blends well with rose and most other oils.

The trees are usually 30 years old before they are ready for oil production. The best sandalwood comes from Mysore, under strict government control; this maintains a high standard. Cheaper oil is produced from Australian sandalwood (a different species). Its aroma and properties are inferior to those of *S. album.* So-called West Indian sandalwood is a totally different species producing what is known as amyris oil. This also has an inferior scent, and is sometimes passed off as true sandalwood by unscrupulous suppliers.

One small drop of true sandalwood oil on your wrist will last for at least 24 hours (don't wash!).

Methods of use • Bath, compress, essence burner and inhalations, massage oil or lotion.

Healing effects • (Antidepressant, antiseptic, antispasmodic, aphrodisiac, astringent, cicatrising, expectorant, sedative, tonic.)

Sandalwood has a beautiful aroma and is an important ingredient in many cosmetics and toiletries (for men as well as women). It has a healing effect on many types of skin problem, especially acne (the oil is both antiseptic and slightly astringent). I have found this oil to be one of the most effective in the treatment of sore throats, bronchitis and urinary infections.

Sandalwood has a remarkable soothing effect on the mind and spirit. It helps calm worries and fears, anger and resentment. It is also reputed to be an aphrodisiac. Blended with ylang ylang, it could help pep up your love-life!

Sandalwood may be considered safe to use throughout pregnancy.

TEA-TREE 🌢 *(Melaleuca alternifolia)*

The essential oil of tea-tree is obtained from the leaves and twigs of a small tree native to Australia (by steam distillation). It has been used by Aborigines for hundreds of years. The aroma can be described as strong medicinal, harsh, lingering and penetrating. Tea-tree oil has been produced since 1930 from trees cut in the swamps. Because of world demand for this new and exciting oil, young plants are now raised in humid greenhouse conditions and are set out after about eight weeks in plantations of bushes rather than of trees.

The potential of this oil is enormous. It boosts the immune system and can help a whole range of conditions. Harmless, natural and effective, tea-tree is the antiseptic of the future.

Methods of use • Bath, compress, essence burner and inhalations, massage oils and lotions, neat application to minor burns or sores. Add to a bland cream or plain live yogurt for thrush.

Caution • Irritant only to very sensitive skins. Deep inhalation of the neat oil can cause dizziness.

Healing effects • (Action: antifungal, antiseptic, deodorant, mental stimulant.)

Tea-tree oil has a non-toxic germicidal action and can be used for colds and flu, cuts and bites. It is recommended for bacterial or fungal vaginitis, such as candida (thrush). To soothe burning and itching, which are symptoms of these infections, use tea-tree cream (keep this in the refrigerator if cold application is required).

Elderly people often have bad circulation in their legs; the skin becomes very thin and the slightest scratch can become infected and ulcerated. They will find a tea-tree cream or a blend of tea-tree and almond oil very soothing.

Tea-tree helps cure dandruff. Add a few drops to your regular shampoo or buy a brand name tea-tree shampoo. Both shampoo and cream are available from suppliers (for mail-order addresses see p. 223).

Sufferers from halitosis and also heavy smokers will find diluted tea-tree helpful as a mouthwash; alternatively, add a few drops of the oil to toothpaste.

Tea-tree has a stimulating effect on the mind and clears a stuffy head. It is also ideal as a first aid remedy for shock and panic.

In pregnancy, tea-tree may be considered safe to use after four months.

YLANG YLANG 🌸 *(Cananga odorata)*

This essential oil is obtained from the beautiful flowers of a tropical tree. The native name means 'flower of flowers'. The blossoms of this tree can be pink, mauve or yellow, but the best oil comes from the yellow sort. The heavy floral aroma has jasmine undertones and is widely used in perfumes.

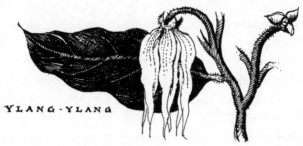

YLANG·YLANG

Ylang ylang comes in different qualities, i.e. Nos 1–4. A lesser quality essential oil is listed separately under the name Cananga (see p. 108).

Methods of use • Bath, essence burner, face oil, massage oils and lotions.

Caution • Used in excess it can cause headaches and nausea. In rare cases it can cause an allergic reaction.

Healing effects • (Antidepressant, antiseptic, aphrodisiac, hypotensive, sedative, tonic.)

Ylang ylang is sometimes called a poor man's substitute for jasmine. It has a quality of its own, however, and should not be compared unfavourably. I find it helpful for people who are angry and frustrated to the extent of causing physical pain (often medically described as symptoms of unknown origin). This oil can also lower high blood pressure and calm palpitations.

A blend of ylang ylang with sandalwood and frankincense is very relaxing, easing tension, anxiety and depression. This particular blend is also good for skin problems and oily complexions.

Ylang ylang is a truly sensual oil and reputedly an aphrodisiac. *In pregnancy, ylang ylang may be considered safe to use after four months.*

CHAPTER 8

Some Further Essential Oils

WHEN YOU HAVE BECOME familiar with using the essential oils detailed in Chapter 7, and have experienced their benefits and versatility, you will want to increase your collection. This chapter is devoted to a further 30 oils, presented a little more briefly. Most of these oils are obtainable from the mail order addresses given on p. 223.

Once again, I must remind you to heed the cautions given in Chapter 5 and those listed against the individual oils detailed below.

ANGELICA ❀ *(Angelica archangelica)*

A member of the Umbelliferae family, angelica is best known in its candied form for culinary use. The essential oil is obtained from the seeds and root.

Methods of use • Bath, essence burner, massage oil or lotion.

Caution • Use in moderation. Avoid during pregnancy.

Healing effects • Helps eliminate a build-up of toxins and excess body fluid. Relieves inflammatory conditions such as gout and arthritis. Alleviates stress-related symptoms such as headache, migraine and mental fatigue. Helps PMT and menopause problems and is a tonic for tired, sluggish skin.

BASIL ❁ *(Ocymum basilicum)*

Essential oil of basil from the Comoro Islands is not recommended for home use because of its high methyl chavicol content (85%). This fact sparked off adverse reports regarding the safety of basil oil. However, basil oil from Egypt has a methyl chavicol content of only 25% which is more acceptable.

Methods of use • Best in an essence burner.

Caution • A skin irritant; use in moderation. Emmenagogue; avoid during pregnancy.

Healing effects • Relieves catarrh, headaches, melancholia, anxiety, insomnia, mental fatigue, poor memory. Uplifting, refreshing, stimulating. Helps dispel resentment, bitterness.

BAY, WEST INDIAN ❁ *(Myrcia acris, Pimenta racemosa)*

The oil does not comes from the bay leaves familiar for its culinary uses but from a different species entirely.

Methods of use • Bath, essence burner, massage lotion.

Healing properties • Stimulates circulation. Traditionally used as a hair tonic (stimulates blood vessels in hair follicles)

– add a few drops of essential oil to your shampoo or conditioner. It can lift depression and sometimes helps rheumatic pain.

BENZOIN 🌿 *(Styrax benzoin)*

Extracted from a tree resin, then dissolved in solvent. It has been used for thousands of years as an incense in magic and rituals. Benzoin is obtainable as a tincture known as Friar's balsam.

Methods of use • Bath, inhalation. Blends well with frankincense in an essence burner.

Healing effects • Sedative and expectorant, it is good for bronchitis and sore throats. Stimulates peripheral circulation and is beneficial for sensitive red skin.

In pregnancy, benzoin may be considered safe to use after four months.

BLACK PEPPER 🌿 *(Piper nigrum)*

A spicy oil, typical of peppercorns in aroma.

Caution • Can irritate sensitive skin. Use in moderation.

Methods of use • Bath , massage oil.

Healing effects • Warming (increases peripheral circulation), stimulates bowels and aids digestion. Eases arthritis and muscular aches and pains. Good after sports activity.

CARDAMOM ❧ *(Ellettaria cardamomum)*

The cardamom plant belongs to the same family as ginger. The aroma of the essential oil is warm and spicy.

Methods of use • As a spice it is used in cooking. The essential oil can be used in the bath or in a massage oil.

Caution • Can irritate sensitive skin.

Healing effects • Helps indigestion and excessive wind. Warming and soothing yet also a stimulant, it relieves headaches, mental fatigue and debility.

Cardamom may be considered safe to use throughout pregnancy.

CANANGA ❧ *(Cananga odorata)*

Cananga comes from the flowers of the same species of tree as ylang ylang (see p. 103), but is of a lesser quality and named differently. Nevertheless, its sweet floral aroma is pleasantly similar to ylang ylang, though it is less heavy. It has similar therapeutic uses.

CINNAMON LEAF ❧ *(Cinnamomum zeylanicum)*

The oil distilled from the leaves is not the same as that from the bark. The two have rather different aromas. Cinnamon bark oil has the traditional spice aroma, while the oil from the leaves is spicy with clove undertones. Cinnamon leaf is best used in an essence burner. Cinnamon bark is one of the oils not recommended for home use (see p. 58).

Essential oil of cinnamon leaf blended with sweet orange makes a delightful aroma to burn at Christmas-time.

Methods of use • Essence burner or inhalation only.

Caution • Very irritating to the skin. In pregnancy, avoid until after seven months, and then use in an essence burner only.

Healing effects • Stimulates the mental faculties. Uplifting and refreshing. It alleviates nasal congestion and bronchial catarrh – treat colds with inhalations.

CLOVE ❧ *(Eugenia caryophyllata)*

The oil is distilled from the flower buds and has the distinctive clove aroma.

Methods of use • Bath, inhalant, essence burner, massage oil. Use neat, on cotton wool, for toothache.

Caution • Can irritate sensitive skins. Avoid during pregnancy.

Healing effects • Analgesic, antispasmodic and expectorant. Stimulates the digestive tract. Eases dyspepsia, diarrhoea and bronchial catarrh. Clove has been used for centuries to relieve toothache.

CITRONELLA ❧ *(Cymbopogon nardus)*

This essential oil comes from an aromatic grass closely related to lemongrass (see p. 113). It has a very pleasant, fresh, sweet, lemony aroma. It is mainly used as an air freshener – it kills unpleasant odours (household or animal) – but it can also be used as a disinfectant.

Methods of use • Essence burner.

Healing effects • Antiseptic, deodorant.

CORIANDER 🌿 *(Coriandrum sativum)*

A warm and spicy oil distilled from the ripe aromatic fruits of the coriander plant.

Methods of use • Bath, essence burner, massage oil.

Caution • Use in moderation. Avoid during pregnancy.

Healing effects • Aids digestion and eases muscular aches and pains. Makes a very relaxing bath. Reputed to be an aphrodisiac.

DILL 🌿 *(Anethum graveolens)*

Dill is well known for its culinary uses. The seeds are used in pickling cucumbers and for flavouring sauces and fish dishes; the leaves are used for similar purposes. Dill oil is employed medicinally to combat flatulance, and is used diluted as dill water for the treatment of gripe in young children.

I have no personal experience using this oil in aromatherapy, but it is said to be useful for children's digestive troubles. Massage the tummy in a clockwise direction – this follows the natural movement of the bowel – and also massage the back. For babies, use 1 drop of dill in 20 ml of base oil.

Dill may be considered safe to use throughout pregnancy.

GALBANUM ❧ *(Ferula galbaniflua)*

Galbanum is distilled from the gum-resin of a plant of the Umbelliferae family that grows in Iran and the Levant. The aroma is warm and spicy but also fresh and leafy. It has been used as an incense for thousands of years. In the perfume industry, galbanum is used as a fixative, i.e. the perfumes are made long-lasting.

Methods of use • Bath, compress, essence burner, inhalant, massage oil or lotion.

Healing effects • Galbanum is useful to alleviate inflamed skin conditions – pustules and boils. It has also been found to relieve rheumatism and gout, muscular strains and respiratory problems.

Use galbanum in an essence burner as an aid for meditation. It is spiritually uplifting and helps to increase awareness.

In pregnancy, galbanum may be considered safe to use after four months.

GINGER ❧ *(Zingiber officinale)*

Distilled from the dried rhizomes, the essential oil has a fresh, woody aroma.

Methods of use • Bath, essence burner, gargle for sore throats, massage oil.

Caution • Use sparingly. May irritate sensitive skins.

Healing effects • Antiseptic, stimulating and warming to the system, ginger is used for colds, rheumatism, muscular aches and pains and nausea. It can also help to relieve nervous tension.

In pregnancy, ginger may be considered safe to use after four months.

HYSSOP ❧ *(Hyssopus officinalis)*

This essential oil, from the leaves of the herb, has a warm, penetrating aroma with camphoraceous undertones.

Methods of use • Bath, essence burner, inhalant, massage oil (blends well with citrus oils).

Caution • Avoid during pregnancy or if epileptic. Use in moderation.

Healing effects • Warming to the system, and opens breathing channels. It is used to treat respiratory problems such as asthma, colds and flu, bronchitis, hay fever and sinusitis. Good for bruises. Helps regulate blood pressure.

JUNIPER BERRY ❧ *(Juniper communis)*

The essential oil extracted from juniper berries smells like gin.

Methods of use • Bath, essence burner, massage oils and lotions (blends well with lavender).

Caution • Use in moderation. Avoid altogether during pregnancy or if suffering from kidney disease.

Healing effects • Diuretic; helps to reduce cellulite and excessive fluid in the tissues. Reduces uric acids and toxins in the system, easing gout, rheumatism, arthritis, and muscular aches and pains. Heals skin ailments, weeping eczema, dermatitis, psoriasis and acne. Calming to the nervous system.

LAVANDIN ❧ *(Lavandula hybrid)*

The essential oil known as lavandin comes from a hybrid between the common lavender *(L. angustifolia)* and *L. latifolia,* sometimes known as spike lavender.

Lavandin oil is very similar to lavender oil in aroma, though slightly harsher (more camphoraceous) and woody sweet. Commercially, it is used in soaps and low cost toiletries.

Methods of use • Bath, inhalation, massage oil, shampoos and hair rubs.

Healing effects • Similar to those of lavender though less powerful. Notably, it appears to be less sedative and versatile. It can be useful if the other properties of lavender are needed without a sedative effect.

Add lavandin to shampoos and hair tonics to promote hair growth.

LEMONGRASS ❧ *(Cymbopogen citratus, and C. flexuosus)*

The oil is extracted from a fragrant tropical grass. It has a strong lemonlike aroma. (Do not confuse lemongrass with lemon verbena *(Lippia citriodoria).*

Methods of use • Essence burner, and as a bath or massage oil provided the skin is not sensitive.

Caution • Can be a skin irritant. Try a patch test first (see p. 57), and always dilute well before external application.

Healing effects • Used in an essence burner, lemongrass is a friendly and relaxing fragrance. It clears unpleasant smells from around the house and will remove a heavy atmosphere (usually caused by negative people). Burning the oil on a regular basis builds positive energies.

Lemongrass has been found beneficial in the healing of torn ligaments and strengthens weak areas due to injury. It is excellent used before sporting activities because of its stimulating properties. It also has a toning effect on oily skins.

Try it as an insect repellant.

In pregnancy, lemongrass may be considered safe to use after four months.

MANDARIN 🌸 *(Citrus reticulata)*

This essential oil comes from the fruit peel and smells just like the fruit.

Methods of use • Bath, essence burner, face oil, massage oils and lotions.

Caution • Possibly phototoxic. Do not use on the skin while sunbathing (see p. 56).

Healing effects • Antiseptic, sedative and calming for digestive complaints. Its gentle action makes it suitable for young children; it will calm them when nervous and soothe tummy upsets.

This oil is excellent for skin care, especially problem skins, toning and tightening (try it blended with clary sage).

Mandarin may be considered safe to use throughout pregnancy.

Myrrh 🌺 *(Commiphora myrrha)*

The essential oil of myrrh is distilled from the gum resin of a desert shrub that grows in north-east Africa. Myrrh was used in antiquity as a perfume, incense and medicine.

Methods of use • Bath, essence burner, massage oil or lotion.

Caution • Avoid during pregnancy.

Healing effects • Myrrh restores lost energy to mind and body. I recommend it for people who feel emotionally drained or in a low state of mind. This oil rejuvenates the whole system, especially the skin. As an expectorant, it is useful in coughs, colds and bronchitis. Traditionally, tincture of myrrh is used for mouth ulcers.

Myrrh opens psychic channels and is sometimes used at séances and by clairvoyants when making readings.

Niaouli 🌺 *(Melaleuca viridiflora)*

Closely related to cajuput (see p. 79), though there are some differences in both properties and aroma (warm, camphoraceous).

Methods of use • Bath, essence burner, gargle, inhalant, massage oil or lotion.

Healing effects • Like cajuput and tea-tree, niaouli is a powerful antiseptic yet non-irritant to the skin. For minor burns, use niaouli neat on sterile gauze to disinfect the wound.

Niaouli is a traditional remedy for respiratory troubles – colds, flu, bronchitis, sinusitis and asthma. It is good also for headaches, and combats cystitis and urinary infections.

Stimulating to the circulation, niaouli is warming and comforting, and good for those suffering from rheumatic aches and pains.

It has a stimulating effect on the mental level as well, clearing muddled thoughts.

In pregnancy, niaouli may be considered safe to use after four months.

ORANGE, SWEET ❧ (*Citrus sinensis*)

A deep golden yellow oil expressed from the peel, it has an aroma just like the fruit.

Methods of use • Bath, compress, essence burner, inhalant, massage oil or lotion.

Caution • May irritate sensitive skins. Possibly phototoxic.

Healing effects • Contains vitamins A, B and C, all valuable for skin care. The oil is used in the treatment of common ailments such as colds and flu, bronchial congestion, fluid retention and constipation. It is helpful during PMT and the menopause, easing anxiety or depression. Many find it spiritually uplifting.

Children love orange oil, as they can easily identify the aroma. It is good when they are chesty and will also help them sleep (use a low dilution for babies and very young children).

Sweet orange may be considered safe to use throughout pregnancy.

PARSLEY 🌿 *(Petroselinum crispum)*

The essential oil is distilled from the seeds.

Methods of use • Massage oil/lotion.

Caution • Use in moderation only, and not at all during pregnancy (emmenogogue).

Healing effect • Diuretic, useful in infections of the urinary tract. Useful also for poor circulation, dysmenorrhoea, liver troubles and digestive upsets.

PINE 🌿 *(Pinus sylvestris and other Pinus species)*

The Scots pine, *Pinus sylvestris,* is a native of northern Europe. The oil is extracted from the needles. (The oil of the dwarf pine *P. pumilio* is regarded as hazardous.)

Methods of use • Bath, essence burner, inhalant, massage oil (used in blends).

Caution • Can cause skin irritation. In pregnancy, avoid until after seven months.

Healing effects • A strong antiseptic, oil of pine is most frequently used in the treatment of respiratory infections – colds, flu, bronchitis, sinusitis. It eases rheumatic aches and pains and stimulates the circulation.

ROSEWOOD ❀ *(Aneba roseaodora)*

This essential oil is obtained from the wood chippings from a tree found in Brazil. Unfortunately, the constant felling of this tree for its wood is depleting the rainforest. Those of us concerned about the environment might sadly decide to give this oil a miss. The aroma is light and spicy with a hint of rose.

Methods of use • Bath, essence burner, massage oil or lotion.

Healing effects • Rosewood is relaxing, calming, soothing, yet uplifting – a comforting oil. It helps to clear headaches and is a gentle toner for the skin. On the mind, it has a soothing and calming effect and is specially recommended for anxiety and stress in young children.

In pregnancy, rosewood may be considered safe to use after four months.

SPANISH SAGE ❀ *(Salvia lavendulaefolia)*

Common sage *(Salvia officinalis)* is not recommended for home use. Spanish sage, however, is much less toxic and its qualities are otherwise very similar. It has a camphoraceous, herby, slightly medicinal aroma.

Methods of use • Bath, essence burner and inhalations, massage oil.

Caution • Use in moderation, and not at all during pregnancy or if epileptic.

Healing effects • (Anti-inflammatory, antiseptic, astringent, diuretic, emmenagogue, expectorant, nerve tonic, stimulant, general tonic.)

Sage restores energy to the whole system, relieving stress and tension. It is a useful remedy for period pain, menopause problems, hormone imbalances, fluid retention, rheumatic aches and pains, sore throats and tonsilitis.

Sage is mentally restorative, helping to dispel lethargy. Use it when you need to make important decisions.

TAGETES ❦ *(Tagetes minuta)*

An oil with a powerful, sweet aroma derived from a small annual plant with bright yellow flowers (related to the French marigold of summer flowerbeds).

Methods of use • Essence burner, massage oil or lotion.

Caution • Can irritate sensitive skins; use in moderation and not at all if there is a tendency to dermatitis, eczema or psoriasis. Do not be tempted to take tagetes internally. In pregnancy, avoid until after seven months and then only in moderation.

Healing effects • Tagetes is chiefly used as a remedy for hard skin, e.g. on the heels, balls of the feet and around elbows and knees. For normal or mature skin, use a low dilution (i.e. 2 drops per 50 ml base) once a week.

Mentally, tagetes has a cheerful, stimulating effect. It clears the mind and lifts the spirits. Blended with basil and used in an essence burner, it helps concentration.

TANGERINE ❦ *(Citrus nobilis)*

See Mandarin (p. 114).

THYME 🌿 *(Thymus vulgaris, and possibly other thyme species)*

The species of thyme most used for the distillation of essential oil is *Thymus vulgaris*, otherwise known as the garden thyme, and the one extensively used in the kitchen.

Methods of use • Bath, compress, essence burner, gargle, hair rinse, massage oil or lotion, mouthwash.

Caution • Can irritate sensitive skin. In pregnancy, avoid until after seven months.

Healing effects • An invaluable antiseptic and traditionally used for the treatment of respiratory infections. Try it as a gargle for sore throats.

Thyme stimulates the circulation, relieves rheumatic aches and pains and strengthens the immune system. It will help dispel both physical and mental fatigue, and also depression and insomnia.

VETIVER(T) 🌿 *(Vetiveria zizanoides)*

This oil comes from an aromatic grass related to lemongrass. Its aroma can be described as rich, heavy, woody, earthy.

Methods of use • Bath, essence burner, massage oil.

A very relaxing oil that helps relieve anxiety, shock, panic, hysteria and fatigue. Excellent for the skin (blends well with mandarin oil).

In pregnancy, vertiver may be considered safe to use after four months.

VIOLET 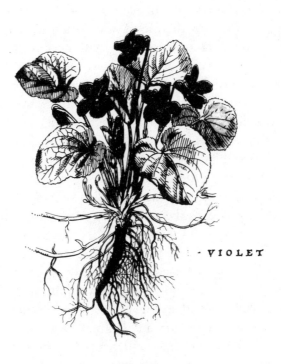 *(Viola odorata)*

An absolute is obtained from the leaf and from the flowers. Violet has antiseptic and expectorant properties – a syrup made from the flowers is traditionally used for coughs and colds. Aromatherapists use the absolute to help relieve kidney problems and skin infections, acne and eczema. It is said to stimulate poor circulation and ease the symptoms of rheumatism.

In pregnancy, violet may be considerd safe to use after four months.

- VIOLET

CHAPTER 9

Massage for Everyone

MASSAGE is one of the oldest forms of treatment. It has a therapeutic effect on the blood and lymph circulation, the nervous system, the respiratory system, and on the muscles and other soft tissues. It encourages the body's ability to heal itself, by restoring free movement to the nutritive fluids. Pressure and stretching push stale fluids away, making room for fresh fluids to take their place. An increased flow of blood increases the supply of oxygen to the tissues.

Massage enables toxins and the breakdown products of inflammation to be more speedily eliminated from the body tissues. Muscles become firmer and more elastic, and skin tone is enhanced with the stimulation of the circulation. The resulting increase of sebum nourishes the skin, and dead cells at the surface are rubbed off, encouraging skin renewal.

The type of massage used today by professional practitioners is mainly Swedish massage, although this does not apply to aromatherapy. Professional aromatherapists study massage techniques in depth. However, the simple soothing massage movements described in this chapter are easy to learn and perfectly suitable for home use.

Massage has a pronounced effect on the psyche. It soothes and calms, creating a feeling of warmth and security. Some people are reminded of babyhood and being held and cherished by their mother. Most babies are continually touched, held and hugged and their bodies rubbed and stroked with oils and creams. Of course the more unfortunate babies, such as the Rumanian orphans, have lacked loving touch and suffered drastic consequences. I'm sure that if everyone received and gave massage regularly we would all be much happier and less aggressive.

Regardless of age, massage can be of help in numerous ailments. In particular, it alleviates tension and fatigue – muscular or mental – aches and pains, strained muscles, stiff joints, arthritis, rheumatism, fibrositis, lumbago (unless very painful) and sciatica, headaches, depression, stress and shock.

You don't have to be ailing to enjoy or benefit from massage. If you have treatment on a regular basis your general health will be greatly improved and maintained.

Generally speaking, in Britain at least, massage is considered a luxury rather than a necessity – a special treat. This attitude is unfortunate as massage is so beneficial. Once a week is best, and certainly once a month cannot be considered excessive. Expense may be a problem, of course. The solution is for one or two members of the family to learn the basic movements, then the whole family can have regular massage.

Family massage improves relationships, bringing you closer together. It could well restore warmth to a marriage that might be failing through lack of touch. Massage is a unique way of communicating without words.

I would recommend taking a beginners' course in basic massage, but if that is not possible there are a number of good books available on the subject. Before you attempt any form of massage, however, there are certain cautions to note.

Do not massage in the following circumstances:

- infectious skin conditions, e.g. impetigo, or around boils or abscesses
- areas where there is an undiagnosed lump or tumour
- cancer cases, unless terminal
- varicose veins
- phlebitis
- thrombosis
- serious heart conditions
- swollen ankles resulting from kidney or heart conditions
- over heavily bruised or broken skin
- fever

NB Special advice on massage during pregnancy is given on pp. 145–46, and on labour on pp. 151–52.

A Simple Massage Procedure

Let us suppose you wish to massage your partner. Here are some easy-to-follow instructions for a very simple basic massage to relax tension and promote sleep.

First of all, make sure the room is warm and quiet with soft lighting (try candle-light). Choose some soft, soothing music. Take the telephone off the hook and keep the children out of the room until it is their turn. If the weather is cool, keep your partner wrapped in blankets; if it is warm, use a light towel or nothing.

Your partner can either lie on the floor or on a large table. Use a duvet, small mattress or strip of foam underneath for comfort. If you are using the floor and kneeling by your partner's side, use a soft cushion under your knees. If you are more comfortable working in direct line with the back, straddle across your partner (this suggestion is only for very good friends!). For just a neck or shoulder problem, your partner may simply sit leaning over a table with arms and head on a pillow.

Beforehand, warm the massage oil by standing the bottle in a bowl of hot water for a minute or two. Always oil your hands first; never pour oil directly onto the body.

Start by using effleurage (stroking movements). This is done by placing the palms of your hands at the base of the spine, fingers together, keeping your hands loose and relaxed, and push firmly but gently up the whole length of the spine. Put the pressure alongside the spine rather than directly on it. When you reach the root of the neck, glide your hands outwards over the shoulders. Then stroke gently down the outer sides of the back with the fingertips, bringing them to the base of the spine ready to repeat the whole movement. Effleurage will spread the oil and soothe the nerves. Make sure oil is massaged over the whole of the back. This is a wonderfully relaxing movement for both you and your partner.

When you feel confident with effleurage, fan your hands alternately outwards at either side of the spine, returning to the base of the spine each time.

Massage tension points at the top of the shoulders in the following manner. Rest your fingers on top of the shoulders

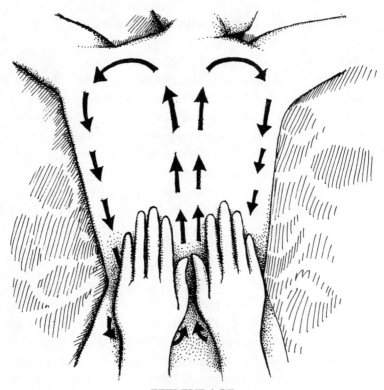

EFFLEURAGE
**Both hands flat on back, fingers loosely together – firm up,
gentle down**

(use them as an anchor rather than squeezing the muscle). With the flat pads of your thumbs firmly massage in outward circular movements – left thumb anticlockwise, right thumb clockwise. Allow your thumbs to be very flexible and cover all the tension areas.

To massage the neck, move your position so that you are facing the neck and head from the side. Place your right

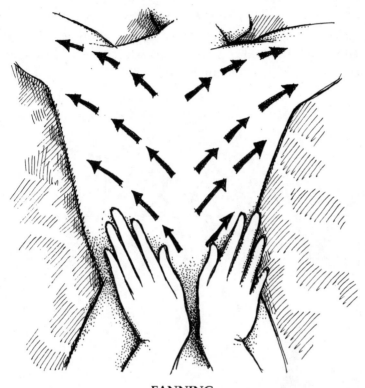

FANNING
Both hands fully on. Stroke outwards, alternating hands

hand over the neck and with your fingers and thumbs firmly massage upwards, using forward and then backward circular movement – as if you were looping string, lifting your fingers on the backward movement.

Start the whole process over again, doing lots of effleurage movements. Finish your massage with long stroking movements down the whole length of the spine, using your palm.

When you have finished, cup your hands over the base of the spine to gather heat and relax for a moment. Slowly lift your hands from the back and cover your partner with a towel or blanket. By now you will hear snoring! I would suggest a 10-minute massage to start with, gradually increasing to 15 or 20 minutes when you are more confident.

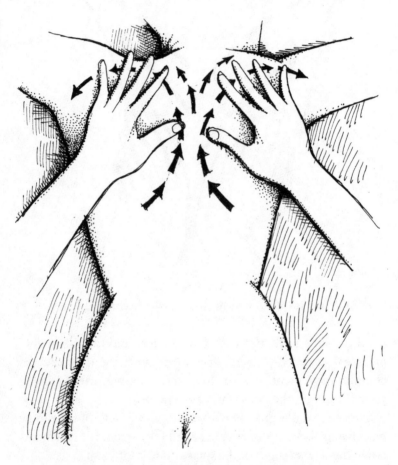

THUMB FRICTION
Use both thumb pads, moving them together alternately

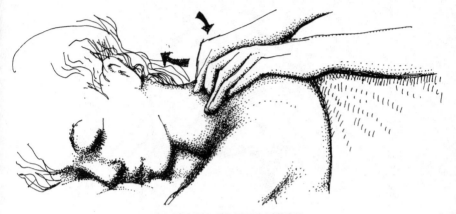

MASSAGE OF THE NECK

Head and Face Massage

To relieve tension, headaches, migraine and sinusitis, use the movements below which are all very easy to perform. Your partner can either lie on the floor or on the bed, with you sitting alongside. Alternatively, he or she can sit on a chair with you standing behind.

For a headache or migraine
Blend in an eggcupful of almond oil 4 drops each of lavender, lemon and peppermint.

Movement 1 • Apply the oil to the forehead and face, stroking outwards with the index, middle and third fingers. Begin at the mid-forehead, stroking towards the temples. Then stroke over the cheeks and under the nose.

129

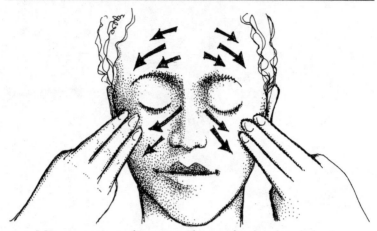

Movement 1: stroke outwards over forehead and cheeks

Movement 2 • Place your hands together, as in prayer, with the base of the hands resting on the forehead. Now firmly stoke outwards across the forehead with the base of each hand, stroking as you do so with the palms and ending with the fingertips on the temples.

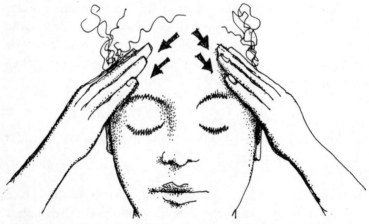

Movement 2: starting with the hands together on the forehead, stroke outwards – base of hands, palms, ending with fingertips

Movement 3 • Stroke in circles around the temples with the index and middle fingers, as in the diagram.

Repeat the above movements some 10 or 12 times or until relief is obtained.

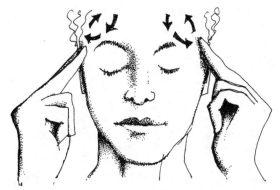

Movement 3: circular stroking of the temples

Scalp massage

Using the pads of all the fingers and the thumbs, knead the scalp using firm, slow movements rotating towards the forehead. This stimulates blood flow, relieving tension and pain.

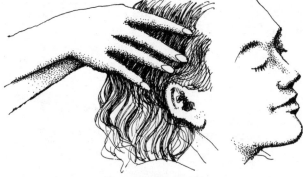

SCALP MASSAGE
Circular movements of the finger and thumb pads

For sinusitis
Blend in an eggcupful of almond oil 4 drops of cedarwood (Virginian), eucalyptus and geranium.

Apply the oil to the forehead and face using **movements 1 and 2** as for headaches (omit movement 3).

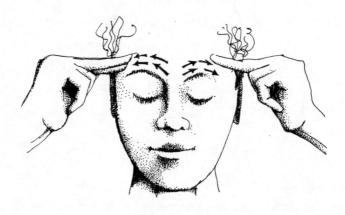

Movement 4

Movement 4 • Using the index and middle fingers, trace a firm line outwards from the centre of the forehead just above the eyebrows. This drains the frontal sinuses.

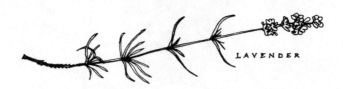

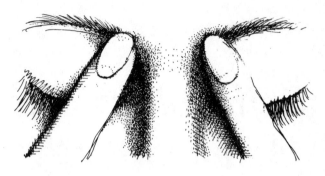

Movement 5

Movement 5 • Locate the pressure point just inside each eye cavity near the beginning of the brow. Using the middle fingers, press and make rotatory movements around it. This drains the ethmoid sinuses.

Movement 6 • Using the index and middle fingers, trace a firm line from the bridge of the nose over the cheek bones. This drains the maxillary sinuses.

Repeat the movements 10 or 12 times or until relief is obtained. Include scalp massage to relieve congestion.

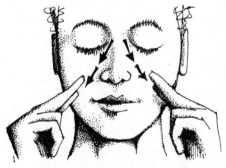

Movement 6

CHAPTER 10

Reflexology and Aromatherapy

DISCOVERED, or – more accurately – rediscovered and introduced to the West by an American surgeon, Dr William Fitzgerald, reflexology has now become well known as a method of diagnosis and treatment by natural means. It has also proven to be a valuable addition to aromatherapy.

Quite a few books have been written on reflexology (also known as zone therapy), so I won't go into it here at great length. Briefly, reflexology is the use of pressure applied to the feet, both the soles and upper parts. The feet resemble a map of the body, and over the years many different charts have been drawn showing how the zones of the feet link with body systems and major organs.

Reflexologists test each zone (called a reflex point) by using a rotatory movement of the thumb. Health problems show up as tender spots on the reflex points. To correct any imbalance, physical or emotional, massage of the reflex point is carried out.

Reflexology works on the body's energy flow, which sometimes becomes blocked. Imbalances can come about for various reasons, e.g. bad eating habits. Blockages create and

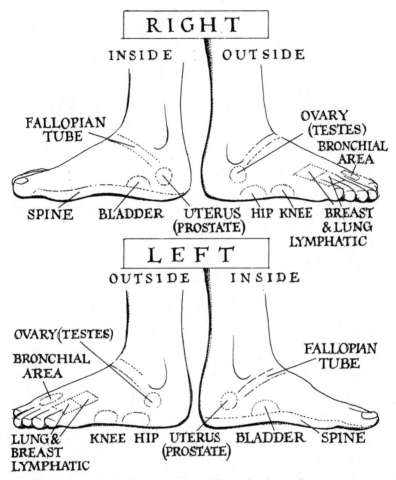

RIGHT

INSIDE   OUTSIDE

FALLOPIAN
TUBE

OVARY
(TESTES)
BRONCHIAL
AREA

SPINE   BLADDER   UTERUS   HIP KNEE   BREAST
(PROSTATE)   &LUNG
LYMPHATIC

LEFT

OUTSIDE   INSIDE

OVARY(TESTES)

BRONCHIAL
AREA

FALLOPIAN
TUBE

LUNG&   KNEE HIP UTERUS   BLADDER   SPINE
BREAST   (PROSTATE)
LYMPHATIC

**Reflex points of the feet (upper and lateral sides) relating to parts
of the body**

overload areas, diminishing or increasing energy behind the
blockage, rather like a traffic jam. As a result, the body then
suffers from low energy, possibly headaches and other aches
and pains, skin problems due to toxicity, and a general

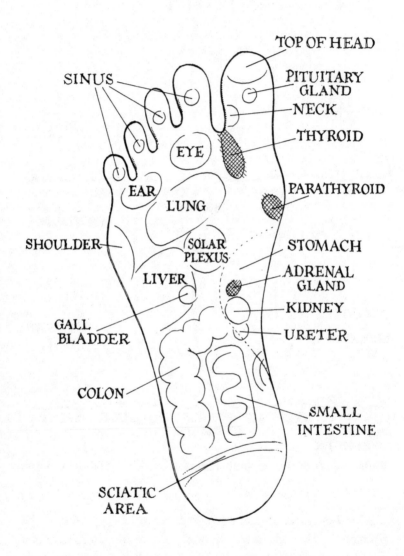

Reflex points of the underside of the right foot

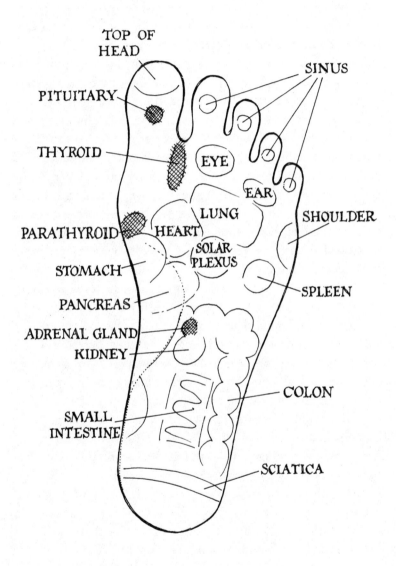

Reflex points of the underside of the left foot

slowing down of vital forces. An excess of energy in the pathways can give rise to inflammation and pain, perhaps leading to more serious, degenerative diseases.

Treating the reflex points helps destroy any energy blocks, thus encouraging the body's own healing capacity to restore harmony and health. The treatment is both relaxing and stimulating; it releases toxins and aids in their elimination.

Reflexology is thought to have originated some 5000 years ago in China, before the discovery of acupuncture and acupressure (therapies used to correct energy balance in the body). In AD 1017, a Dr Wang Wei was teaching students of acupuncture the use of deep pressure on the soles and sides of the feet, with emphasis on the big toe. The feet were massaged whilst the acupuncture needles were in position, channelling extra energy.

Thousands of years ago, before shoes were invented, ancient man felt nature's energies through his feet. The uneven ground would have stimulated reflex points in the soles. We all know how painful walking barefoot on a pebble beach can be – but it's a good way of stimulating the pressure points! You can of course massage your own feet, or ask a friend or relative to do it for you.

Professional aromatherapists often use reflexology as a diagnostic aid and include it in their treatment programme. Reflexology massage, in stimulating the energy flow, aids the absorption of essential oils.

Reflexology can be used to treat all kinds of common ailments. Of course it isn't always possible to visit a qualified therapist, but for minor problems there is a self-help method combining aromatherapy with reflexology.

Self-help Reflexology

A relaxing aromatherapy foot massage

Add 8 drops of lavender or cypress oil to a bowl of comfortably warm water and give it a good swish. Take the telephone off the hook, relax and soak your feet for 15 minutes in the warm, aromatic water. Dry your feet and relax on a sofa or bed, supporting your back with pillows. Meanwhile, use your essence burner with your favourite relaxing oil.

Put your right foot on your left thigh. Massage it using light friction, alternately up and down. Then, using your favourite massage blend, knead and stroke the foot using deep, soothing movements, alternately. Include the ankle, toes and soles. Stretch and pull the feet upwards and outwards.

Massage the foot for 5 minutes, making sure the oils have been absorbed. Rub off any excess oil with a towel or tissue.

With a reflexology chart propped up in front of you, press each reflex point of the foot in turn, starting with the top of the big toe. Note any discomfort (you may already be aware of areas that need attention). Concentrate on the tender areas.

When you have finished, place the left foot on the right thigh and follow the same procedure. In reflexology it is most important to treat both your feet.

Try to set aside some time regularly for your aromatherapy foot massage.

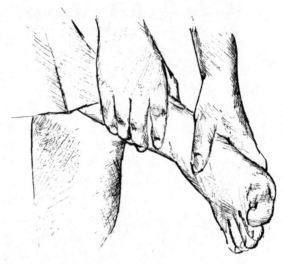

Treating minor ailments

It is possible to treat a specific area of your body with essential oils. (**Caution:** do not attempt to use this method on babies or young children.)

Massage the foot with plain base oil, applying 1 drop of essential oil to the specific reflex point. For example, you could use frankincense to relax the solar plexus. Here are some further examples:

Headache, use 1 drop lavender and 1 drop peppermint on the reflex point on the top of the big toe.

PMT, use 1 drop of cypress on the ovary reflex point.

To release anger, use 1 drop camomile or rose on the liver reflex point.

Carry out the treatment once or twice a week until improvement is felt.

CHAPTER 11

Pregnancy and Afterwards

AROMATHERAPY is an excellent way for a woman to remain relaxed, calm and healthy during pregnancy and in the weeks just after the birth. At this time you tend to be sensitive and very emotional on account of the hormonal changes and adjustments your body is going through. Throughout these months, you should be treated, and treat yourself, as very special.

While pregnancy may be one of the most exciting times of your life, there can be unpleasant problems, fears and worries to cope with. If you are a first-time mother, you may find adjusting to pregnancy difficult and have to deal with mixed emotions. Emotions are passed on to the developing baby in the womb.

There is always an abundance of good advice regarding sensible foods to eat and vitamins to take. And there are warnings about smoking and excessive alcohol intake being dangerous to the growth of the baby. To these warnings one should add that it is very harmful for the foetus to absorb arguments, emotional traumas, shocks, depression, tension and worry. As well as healthy foods and vitamins, the developing child will thrive on love, peace, harmony and relaxation, feelings of warmth and comfort, and, most of all, loving communication, not just from you but from the rest of the family as well.

Fatigue is an obstacle to be overcome during pregnancy, for, whilst this should be considered as a special time, life still tends to go on in the same old way. Work has to be carried out, the home has to be cleaned, shopping, cooking, washing, ironing done, and the whole household organised. The more fortunate ladies have housekeepers, cleaning ladies or au pairs to take care of most of the mundane chores. But the average working mum has to cope mostly alone. If there are older children in the family, they can be a great help (sometimes) and of course so can the husband (if so inclined).

Whatever your lifestyle, aromatherapy can help you. You do not have to endure nervous tension. Ask your family and friends to join in with massage (see p. 145), or have treatment on a regular basis from a qualified therapist at least once a month (better still once a week). Failing that, there is self-help reflexology (see p. 139). All through your pregnancy, as well as having aromatherapy treatments using calming, fortifying and uplifting oils, include relaxation techniques such as meditation.

During pregnancy many irritating health problems can occur. The following are among the most common: backache, constipation, fainting and nausea, insomnia, skin changes, high blood pressure and circulatory problems, such as varicose veins, and swollen legs and ankles due to fluid retention. Most of these respond well to aromatherapy. The treatment of common ailments is dealt with in Chapter 14, but for pregnancy there are special instructions and cautions.

When you are pregnant it is especially important to know how to use essential oils properly. You should use fewer drops than generally recommended. Restrict the use of essential oils in the bath or in massage oils to two or three times a week (unless guided by a qualified practitioner). An essence burner can be used every day, however, because it diffuses the oil considerably.

Certain oils can be harmful to the foetus and should be absolutely avoided – pennyroyal, cedarwood and thuja are considered abortive.

Advice is sometimes conflicting in books on aromatherapy. For example, one author says that rose should not be used because it is a stimulant for the uterus. Another aromatherapist actually recommends rose oil. The wife of a well-known authority actually took rose internally during her own pregnancy. As each oil tends to have a slightly different effect on individuals, there can be no overall directive except against abortive and toxic oils.

Certain oils are emmenagogue, i.e. inducing or increasing menstrual flow. These oils, which include basil, camphor, clary sage, hyssop, marjoram, myrrh, sage and rosemary, can be harmful in early pregnancy, especially if there is a history of miscarriage. Camomile and lavender are mild emmenagogues and are best avoided as well. If the pregnancy is strong and trouble-free, and the mother fit and healthy, there is unlikely to be any risk, though it is best to observe caution all the same. (Even camomile tea is best avoided in early pregnancy.)

If you have miscarried previously, or have been told by your doctor there is some risk, consult a qualified aromatherapist. Also, inform your doctor and midwife that you wish to use aromatherapy.

Suitable Oils

The oils listed below are considered safe for the respective stages of pregnancy but use them in the dilutions recommended in the recipes.

For first four months

The following oils are considered safe: bergamot, cardamom, dill, grapefruit, lemon, mandarin, melissa, orange (sweet), peppermint, spearmint, sandalwood.

After four months

Add these to your repertoire: benzoin, cajuput, cypress, eucalyptus, frankincense, galbanum, geranium, ginger, jasmine, lemongrass, neroli, niaouli, patchouli, petigrain, rose (in face oil), rosewood, tea-tree, vetiver, violet leaf, ylang ylang.

After seven months

You can include, in low dosage and preferably in an essence burner or face oil: camomile, cinnamon leaf (burner only) clary sage, lavender, rose, rosemary (for tiredness and backache), thyme.

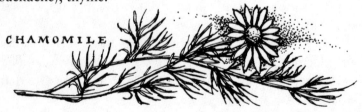

CHAMOMILE

Massage During Pregnancy

To give a relaxation massage to someone in the early months of pregnancy, get her to sit or lean over a table with arms and head on a pillow. Just massage the neck and shoulders. Do not attempt any other massage in the first four months. From the fifth month, massage the shoulders and limbs with the essential oils recommended above. You can also lightly apply oil to the abdomen to prevent stretch marks. During the more advanced stages of pregnancy, concentrate your massage on the shoulders, neck, face and head, limbs, feet and ankles.

Recipes and Treatments

The recipes in this section contain oils that are widely available and not too expensive

The following dilutions are recommended:

Bath, 2–4 drops
Massage oil/lotion, 4–6 drops to 50 ml base
Essence burner, 4–6 drops.

The following recipes are suitable for any stage of pregnancy, including the first four months –

Energy blend for massage or bath oil
Two drops bergamot, 2 drops mandarin.

Relaxing face and body oil
Two drops each of bergamot, sandalwood and mandarin.

Uplifting massage oil
Two drops each of peppermint or spearmint, grapefruit and melissa.

Bath oils
(Add a cup of milk or 1 tablespoon vegetable oil.)

Refreshing: 2 drops mandarin, 2 drops lemon.

Cooling: 4 drops peppermint.

Massage oil/lotion to prevent stretch-marks
Three drops lemon, 3 drops mandarin.

For morning sickness

There is not a lot you can do if you are suffering severely from morning sickness, but the following suggestions may give some relief. Put a few drops of ginger or cardamom oil on your pillow or on a pad of cotton wool by your head at night. In the morning, light your essence burner using 6 drops of peppermint. Also try a cup of herbal peppermint tea, or just plain boiled water, with a plain biscuit.

The following recipes should only be used after four months –

Relaxing face and body oil
Two drops patchouli, 2 drops jasmine, 2 drops lemon.

Or, 3 drops neroli, 3 drops bergamot.

Relaxing massage oil
Two drops each of geranium, ylang ylang and patchouli.
Or, 2 drops frankincense, 4 drops sandalwood.

Uplifting/stimulating massage oil
Two drops each of eucalyptus, ginger and sweet orange.

Bath oils
(Add a cup of milk or 1 tablespoon vegetable oil.)

Relaxing: 2 drops bergamot, 2 drops ylang ylang.
Or, 2 drops geranium, 2 drops patchouli.
Or, 2 drops vetiver, 2 drops neroli.
Or, 2 drops mandarin, 2 drops vetiver.

For fatigue: 2 drops frankincense, 2 drops grapefruit or cypress.

For insomnia: 2 drops bergamot, 2 drops ylang ylang

Refreshing and cooling (also for headaches): 2 drops peppermint, 2 drops lemon.

Backache
For massage oil, blend 3 drops niaouli, 3 drops ginger or cajuput.

Colds and flu
For use in bath and essence burner: 2 drops tea-tree, 2 drops lemon or cajuput.

Cystitis

For massage oil, blend 3 drops sandalwood, 3 drops eucalyptus. Apply to lowest part of the abdomen, over and just above the pubic hair.

Dry skin, psoriasis, eczema

For massage oil/lotion, blend 2 drops each of ylang ylang and sandalwood, and 2 drops of patchouli or neroli. If possible, for the base use almond oil with some wheatgerm oil added to it (a good source of vitamin E).

Insomnia

For massage oil, mix 2 drops bergamot, 2 drops ylang ylang. Massage the face, the region 2 inches below the breast bone (bra line) and the feet (see Chapter 10 on reflexology). The same combination can be used in the bath or essence burner. Or try a few drops of patchouli in your essence burner.

To protect against viral infections

For bath or essence burner: 4 drops tea-tree or lemon.

To protect your home or work environment against infection, regularly vaporise tea-tree oil in an essence burner, and add it to your bathwater if you have been exposed to a virus. German measles (Rubella) and measles are specially dangerous if contracted whilst pregnant.

To prevent stretch marks (after 5 months)

For massage oil/lotion, add 2 drops each of frankincense, sandalwood and lemon. Massage sides of abdomen and tops of legs.

Swollen legs and ankles (fluid retention)
For a massage oil, blend 2 drops each of grapefruit, lemon, and either cajuput or patchouli. Massage using upward movements away from the ankles towards the thighs.

Varicose veins
For a massage oil, blend 4 drops cypress, 2 drops geranium.

Towards the end of the pregnancy, you may try the following –

For fear and anxiety
At the start of and during labour, use the following blend in an essence burner: 3 drops each of clary sage and frankincense, and 3 drops of lavender or camomile.

Compress for during labour
Use two small, soft towels. Lay the compress across the lower abdomen and/or across the vaginal area. To keep the compress warm, use the towels alternately. Add to 2 pints of warm water 15 drops of any of the following oils, either singly or in combination: cajuput, clary sage, jasmine, lavender.

Not Forgetting Father

What about father? He needs his share of relaxation during your pregnancy and afterwards.

For anxious father's bath

The first is a 'knock-out' formula, so don't use this if he is needed for emergencies!

1) 4 drops clary sage, 4 drops sandalwood or vetivert, 3 drops ylang ylang.

2) 4 drops bergamot, 4 drops camomile, 4 drops geranium.

Father's 'pep up' bath

Mix 4 drops peppermint, 4 drops eucalyptus, 4 drops grapefruit.

During Labour

If you are having your baby at home, it will be easy for you to implement an aromatherapy relaxation programme. If, on the other hand, you are going to have your baby in hospital then ask the midwife and nurses to allow you to have your essence burner, compresses, massage oils and cassette player in the delivery room.

Perhaps your husband or boyfriend or another member of the family will be with you during labour. If so, get them to massage your shoulders, neck, arms and hands, legs and feet. Lay on your side and have a very gentle soothing rub on your hips and lower back.

Use frankincense or lemongrass in your essence burner. These purify the air and the psychic atmosphere, so your baby will arrive in surroundings free from negative energies.

If you are very nervous, put some clary sage or lavender on your pillow or on a cotton wool pad and waft it under your nose from time to time.

Pain relief

Try the following recipe for a pain-relieving massage oil/lotion: to 50 ml base oil add 2 drops camomile or lavender, 3 drops cajuput, 2 drops peppermint.

Warm compresses can relax the muscles and very effectively ease pain. Have two soft towels or large flannels to use as compresses. To 2 pints of warm water add 15 drops clary sage. Soak a towel in this, squeeze it out and place on the lower abdomen. Repeat compresses using alternate towels to keep the tummy warm. For extra pain relief, place lavender or jasmine compresses over the pubic area.

To fortify the mind and spirits, in an essence burner, use 4 drops of either frankincense or lemongrass, or 2 drops each galbanum and vetiver

One of my clients inhaled clary sage and lavender from a cotton pad during labour. She said the effect was almost tantamount to gas and air. The midwife was most impressed.

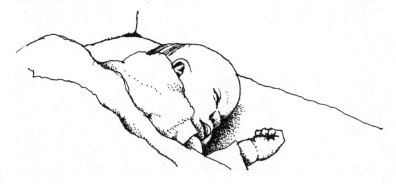

After the Birth

Now your baby has arrived it is still necessary to keep the atmosphere as peaceful and harmonious as possible. He/she will be sensitive to emotional changes and may feel insecure and become fretful.

You have delivered the goods, but your work is only just beginning. Your body has to adjust to getting back to a normal routine and you will need to restore your energy levels – so do keep up your aromatherapy treatments.

Although some women sail through pregnancies and childbirth with little or no emotional change, some suffer dreadfully with post-natal depression. Aromatherapy can be of immense help in this situation.

Do not expose your newborn baby to high doses of essential oils. For the first two weeks, if you want to burn oils for yourself, keep the burner in a separate room.

During the first few weeks you will probably feel rather sensitive. Strong, stimulating oils are not advisable at this time, especially if you are breastfeeding. Use oils such as camomile, cypress, frankincense, geranium, grapefruit, jasmine, lavender, neroli and sandalwood. Keep the number of drops to the minimum, i.e. 2–4 drops in a bath, 4–6 drops in a massage oil.

Note on breast-feeding

As essential oils are absorbed into the body, lactating mothers must not exceed 2–3 drops for a bath and 6–8 drops in 50 ml base oil. Choose from the following: camomile, cedarwood, bergamot, frankincense, geranium, grapefruit, jasmine, mandarin, neroli, rose, sandalwood, ylang ylang.

If using essential oils whilst breast-feeding, remember to drink plenty of water.

To help increase the flow of milk, you could try a massage oil of 10 drops of either fennel or dill to 50 ml base oil. Clean the breasts before feeding.

To restore energy levels

Try this combination: 2 drops frankincense, 2 drops rosemary.

Post-natal depression

To 50 ml base oil, add 4 drops cypress, 2 drops sandalwood. (Cypress helps balance hormones.) Massage the abdomen and solar plexus region.

Or you could try the following oils, either in combination or individually: jasmine, clary sage, rose, melissa, sandalwood. Use the oils on your pillow at night, or in an essence burner.

Keep your diet light and free from heavy, spicy foods. Cut down on salt and sugar intake. Eat plenty of fruit and green vegetables and cut out all red meat, especially pork – become at least semi-vegetarian for a while. Take plenty of water, fresh air and some gentle exercise. Try to think positively about your life. You have just given birth to a new human being who needs love, protection and emotional harmony.

Essential Oils for Young Babies

In India, newborn babies are massaged with olive oil. This strengthens their limbs and nourishes the skin. If your baby's skin is dry, massage with almond oil mixed with a little olive oil. To 50 ml of this base oil, add 1 drop of lavender or Roman camomile.

Mineral oil is not recommended as it is drying to the skin.

For babies of 2 weeks up to 2 months, the following essential oils are suitable: camomile (Roman and German), dill, eucalyptus, lavender, neroli, rose (otto).

For babies over the age of 2 months, bergamot, fennel, frankincense, ginger, niaouli, sweet orange, patchouli, petitgrain, rosemary, rosewood, sandalwood and ylang ylang may be added.

Dilutions for babies aged 2 weeks to 2 months: bath, 1 drop; massage oil, 2 drops to 50 ml base oil. *For babies aged 2 months and up to 2 years*, these amounts can be increased by 1 drop. (A table of dilutions for babies and children is on p. 160.)

Babies should not receive essential oils every day. Two or three times a week is the maximum, whether by essence burner, bath or a massage oil. On the other days, massage your baby with a bland oil, such as almond or apricot.

If you wish to use an essence burner, it must have a deep enough dish to hold water for two hours' vaporising – do not use neat essential oils on a source of heat for young babies. Two drops should be the maximum. Should you not have a suitable essence burner, an alternative would be a bowl of hot water; add two or three drops.

Keep the vaporised oils away from baby's face and head –

direct inhalation will prove too much for such a delicate mite.

A relaxing bath for baby
Use 1 drop of either lavender or Roman camomile. Before adding the essential oil to the water, put in 15 ml almond oil or creamy milk. Swish the water thoroughly. Then add baby!

Colds and snuffles
Place a bowl of hot water near the cot and add 1 drop lavender, 1 drop eucalyptus or tea-tree. An essence burner could be used if of a suitable type.

Colic
Up to 2 months: To 50 ml base oil add 3 drops of dill.
From 2 months: To 50 ml base oil add 2 drops dill and 1 drop fennel. Massage the tummy in circular movements, and also massage the back.

Constipation
Up to 2 months: Try a massage oil containing 1 drop rosemary and 1 drop sweet orange or fennel in 50 ml base. Massage the abdomen in a clockwise direction.

Diarrhoea
Over 2 months: Blend 1 drop ginger, 1 drop lemon or camomile and use as a compress. A massage oil can also be made with this blend (add to 50 ml base oil), but apply gently – massage will stimulate the bowel.

Disturbed sleep
To 50 ml base oil add 1 drop rose and 1 drop camomile or neroli.
Over 2 months: Vaporise 2 drops frankincense, or 1 drop lavender, 1 drop bergamot in a bowl of water or suitable essence burner. For a bath, add 1 drop each of petitgrain and ylang ylang.

Skin problems (dry patches, rash)
Up to 2 months: To 40 ml almond oil add 10 ml virgin olive oil or apricot kernel oil. Then add either 2 drops neroli or 2 drops German camomile.
Over 2 months: Make a massage oil consisting of 1 drop bergamot and 2 drops lavender or patchouli to 50 ml base. For a bath, use 2 drops sandalwood.

Breathing difficulties/asthma
Up to 3/4 months: Frankincense is marvellous for asthma, as it relaxes the chest muscles and calms anxiety which in turn affects breathing. Also try vaporising lavender and sweet orange. For a massage oil, to 50 ml sweet almond/apricot kernel oil add 1 drop lavender, 1 drop sweet orange. Massage the chest and back. The same mixture can be added to the bathwater.

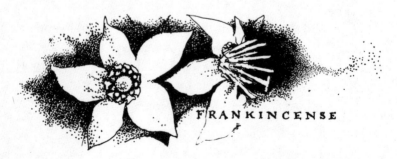

FRANKINCENSE

As Your Baby Grows

Continue to use aromatic oils for your baby as he/she grows. In the following chapter guidelines and recipes are given for children of all ages.

Relaxing massage oil for babies aged 3 months and over

To 50 ml sweet almond/apricot oil add 1 drop mandarin/tangerine, 2 drops rosewood or neroli.

Or, 2 drops Roman camomile, 1 drop mandarin/tangerine or sandalwood.

CHAPTER 12

From Tots to Teens

AT THE END of the last chapter, instructions were given on the use of aromatherapy for young babies. As your child grows, aromatherapy can continue to help with many of his/her health problems, but of course always obtain medical advice whenever necessary.

Encourage children, especially if they are receiving essential oils regularly, to drink plain still water (bottled or filtered). This not only helps excretion of toxins from the body but removes essential oils from the bloodstream.

Essential Oils for Children

The following oils are considered suitable for children from 6 months to 10 years (but do a patch test first):

Bergamot, cajuput, camomile, dill, eucalyptus, frankincense, geranium, ginger, jasmine, lavender, lemon, mandarin/tangerine, neroli, sweet orange, patchouli, peppermint, petitgrain, rose, rosemary (in moderation), rosewood, sandalwood, tea-tree, violet, ylang ylang.

The recommended amount of each essential oil in the recipes given in this chapter is the maximum you should use for a child aged 6 months to 2 years (unless otherwise indicated). For older children, increase the number of drops according to the table on page 160.

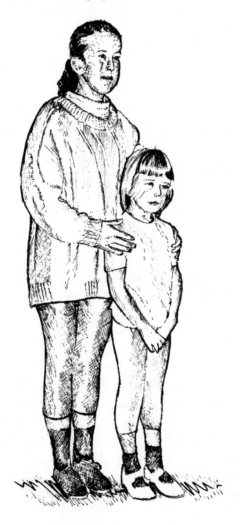

Essential Oil Quantities Table

Child's age	Bath Maximum total of drops (first dissolve in milk)	Massage oil Maximum total of drops in 50 ml base oil
2 weeks– 2 months	1	2
2 months– 2 years	2–3	3
2–5 years	3–4	3–5
5–10 years	4–5	5–6
10–15 years	6–8	8–10

Recipes for Children's Common Ailments

Acne

Wash the face at least twice a day, and I suggest you use a pure honey-based soap obtainable in health food shops. Rinse very well. Every other day use a gentle facial scrub until the condition begins to clear, then twice a week. Three times a week use a face mask of plain live yogurt (it kills bacteria).

The face should not be steamed as this might spread infection. The same can happen if the spots are touched or squeezed (this damages the tissue and can leave a scar).

When pustules are very bad, use a cotton bud and put neat lavender oil carefully on each one. If they need to be popped, pull the skin on either side of the spot apart using cotton wool pads, rather than squeeze – if the spot is ready to pop it will release the pus. Apply neat lavender or tea-tree oil to the spot to prevent further infection.

As well as using the scrubs and yogurt, acne can betreated with a lotion: to 50 ml base oil/lotion, add 8 drops tea-tree, 5 drops lavender, 5 drops lemongrass (if there is an adverse skin reaction use lemon instead). Use this once a day until the condition improves, then every other day.

Asthma

If the child is very sensitive, essential oils may aggravate asthma. More often than not, however, they help enormously, both with opening up the breathing channels and relieving anxiety. To be on the safe side, introduce essential oils slowly and in small doses to start with.

Recommended oils for young children up to 8 years are: lavender, sweet orange, eucalyptus, frankincense and tea-tree. For children over 8 years of age you may include cajuput, hyssop (unless epileptic), lemon, peppermint and pine. Experiment to see which oil (or oils) suits your child best. Try them in the bath, in an essence burner, or as a massage oil for the chest and back.

Athlete's foot

For children of all ages, use a bland lotion or cream base and to 50 ml add 20 drops of tea-tree oil. A ready-prepared tea-tree cream is obtainable through suppliers. Rub on the affected area before bedtime. Alternatively, dab on neat tea-tree oil with a cotton bud.

A foot bath used regularly will relieve symptoms and prevent re-infection: 20 drops of tea-tree in a bowl of warm water. Dry the feet thoroughly.

Add tea-tree oil to unperfumed, purified talc and use during the day. You must keep the feet dry and free from perspiration (cotton socks should be worn).

Colds, flu and breathing difficulties
For a massage oil for chest and back, to 50 ml base oil add 3 drops tea-tree, 2 drops eucalyptus, 2 drops lavender.

In the bath, use 2 drops tea-tree, 2 drops lavender.
For essence burner: eucalyptus.

When using an essence burner in a child's bedroom, keep it out of reach of inquisitive hands.

Constipation
Massage oil: to 20 ml base oil add 1 drop each of fennel, lavender and rosemary. Massage the abdomen gently in a clockwise direction – this follows the natural peristalsis action of the intestines.

Diarrhoea
For a massage oil for tots up to 2 years, to 50 ml base add 2 drops camomile and 1 drop ginger. For older children, you can also use essential oils such as lavender, lemon and sandalwood. Massage very gently. If the diarrhoea is severe, consult your doctor.

Disturbed sleep

Lavender in an essence burner in the child's bedroom will help. Also try 2 drops frankincense in the bathwater, or a massage oil with lavender, rose and/or clary sage.

Headache due to anxiety

Around exam times children are often stressed and anxious. Indeed, the whole atmosphere of the house can be quite strained. Use an essence burner with peppermint, lemon, marjoram and lavender, in equal amounts. The same combination can be used in a bath.

Period pains and irregularities

For many young girls this is a source of much distress every month.

To relieve pain, make up a massage oil consisting of half an eggcupful of almond oil and 2 drops each of cajuput, camomile, peppermint and clary sage. Massage the lower abdomen with the oil, then give her a comforting hot-water bottle wrapped in a towel to hug against the tummy.

If the pain is really bad, she should sip a cup of hot water containing one drop of peppermint oil.

To help prevent period pains and to regulate an irregular menstrual cycle, try the following massage oil/lotion once a day over the 10 days before the period: 3 drops cypress, 3 drops lavender and 4 drops camomile in 50 ml base. (For the adult formula, see p. 208.)

Swollen glands

Over the affected area, gently apply an oil, lotion or compress containing 3 drops frankincense, 3 drops lavender. Repeat three times a day until improvement.

Tummy-ache (from anxiety or over-eating)
To 20 ml base oil add 1 drop camomile, 1 drop cajuput, 1 drop peppermint. Massage the back and the tummy (in a clockwise direction).

❧ CHAPTER 13 ❧

Aromatherapy for Senior Citizens

Growing old does not automatically mean becoming ill. Learning to be relaxed and to cope with the ageing process depends very much on your mental outlook. If you expect everything will wear out, break down and fall off, then you will not be disappointed – you will have an old age rife with physical problems.

Maybe you have been suffering from a chronic condition and have been told there is no cure. Do not sink into acceptance, or decide to learn to live with it. Take up the challenge and seek a way to improve your situation. Even if you are unable to find a total cure, the change in outlook will at least make the symptoms easier to bear.

People of any age find it difficult to change after they have become set in their ways. But the first thing you must do in advancing years is to stop using the expression 'I am getting old'. Change this to 'I am maturing in the pattern of my youth' (a quote from Dr Stuart Grayson, lecturer and writer).

Learn to relax the reins on the amount of jobs done in a day, and cease worrying about niggling matters – worry does not cure anything. Allow more time for rest and recreation. Embrace this period of your life as something precious and beautiful. Think of all the wisdom you can pass on to those who will welcome your experience.

Nowadays people generally live longer and are more active in old age than ever before. As you get older, you may feel that now your family has grown up, and moved away perhaps, you no longer have a purpose in life. Rubbish! You are valuable and needed, and aromatherapy is an area where you can learn to help yourself and your friends. Learn how to use essential oils and, if you are physically active, basic massage skills. Massage your husband/wife, friends, family or neighbours. This can be a very rewarding occupation.

I have taught many people over 60 the fundamentals of aromatherapy and massage, and they have been delighted with their new-found skills. Something special has been added to their lives; they've felt stimulated, too. The learning process brought about changes within their lives they did not think possible. For example, one elderly couple who attended a beginners' class wrote to me to thank me for bringing them much closer together; they felt more relaxed and less irritable with each other.

Aromatherapy can help the elderly in many ways. Use essential oils at home to alleviate aches and pains, arthritic and rheumatic conditions, feelings of loneliness and sadness, depression, respiratory problems, and general tiredness and fatigue.

When using essential oils in the bath, always use a slip mat or side support to prevent accidents.

Essence burners in the house will keep you feeling cheerful and mentally alert. They will also help you to sleep peacefully (but blow out the candle before going to sleep).

You can apply essential oils – in massage oils, lotions or compresses – to your painful arthritic joints (if you have any). Whenever applying body oil or lotion to the feet, remember to wipe off the excess and put slippers on immediately, to avoid slipping on the floor.

Why not run an aromatherapy self-help group in your community? Encourage a communal charge to cover the cost of oils and, perhaps, a massage couch. You will need at least six inexpensive oils to start with (obviously there must be an initial outlay, but you will find the oils last a long time).

Elderly husbands and wives can help each other with their various problems, massaging each other for aching backs, stiff necks and shoulders, painful knees and ankles. Apart from the relief of pain, this encourages *closeness and comfort* through touch, which I'm sad to say sometimes becomes neglected over the years. It will bring you closer together. If you live alone, ask one of your children to massage you, or ask a friend to rub your neck and shoulders.

A Regular Routine

If you are fortunate enough to be able to have a massage regularly, either by visiting a masseuse or asking a therapist to visit you, make it one of your regular routines. Massage will certainly help to loosen up your creaky bits, ease your aches and pains, pep up your circulation, stretch and relax your muscles, and soothe the nervous system. It will also help regulate your blood pressure.

If you can employ a mobile therapist, have a group massage session once a week or fortnight. Ask your friends, family or neighbours to come in and share the costs. The more timid ones will then be encouraged to have a go. Make it a social occasion and encourage participation on a regular basis.

After having your first massage, you may feel a little stiff initially, because the stimulation of the circulation releases toxins. Muscles that have not been receiving enough oxygen or fresh blood become sluggish. After the first two massage treatments you will begin to wonder why you waited so long – it is the very best kind of medicine and combined with essential oils will give you a new lease of life.

Some Essential Oils for the Youthfully Matured

(Remember not to use rosemary if suffering from high blood pressure.)

Basil and rosemary: to alleviate mental fatigue.

Cajuput, eucalyptus and lavender: for arthritis and rheumatic conditions.

Camomile and lavender: to ease aches and pains, muscular spasms and cramp.

Black pepper and juniper: for general aches and pains and muscular stiffness.

Marjoram: for aches and pains, and feelings of loneliness and grief.

Rosemary: for bad circulation.

Sandalwood and frankincense: to enhance spirituality.

The recipes below I have found to be very effective for specific conditions. The quantities of essential oils have been kept to the minimum to ensure the safety of delicate skin. But if relief is not obtained, increase the amounts to a maximum of 25 drops per 50ml base oil. Remember, when making massage oils or lotions, that 50 ml is approximately equivalent to 2 tablespoons.

For baths, don't forget to add 1 cup of milk to comfortably warm water before adding the recommended essential oils.

Bath to ease arthritis and rheumatism
Add 3 drops each of camomile, lavender, marjoram.
Or, 3 drops cajuput, 3 drops eucalyptus, 3 drops lavender or pine.

Bath for general aches/muscular stiffness
Add 5 drops lavender, 3 drops juniper, 3 drops rosemary.
Or, 3 drops each of eucalyptus, marjoram and camomile.

Bath for general fatigue

Add 3 drops each of frankincense, grapefruit and rosemary. Avoid rosemary if you have high blood pressure.

Massage oil/compress for painful arthritic joints

To 50 ml peanut (arachis) oil base add 5 drops each of cajuput, camomile and lemon.

Peanut oil is specially good for arthritis.

If the joints are swollen and inflamed, use the same combination for a compress. Add the essential oils to 1 pint of warm water. Soak a soft flannel or small towel, and apply to the affected joint. Keep the compress warm (see p. 67).

Massage oil for lower back pain (lumbago)

To 50 ml base oil/lotion add 5 drops each of black pepper, lemon and juniper.

Or, 5 drops each of ginger, niaouli and lavender.

Massage oil for general muscular aches and pains

To 50 ml base, preferably peanut (arachis) oil, add 5 drops of camomile, 5 drops lavender and 5 drops of either black pepper, eucalyptus, marjoram or rosemary.

Ulcerated varicose veins

Add 20 drops lavender or tea-tree to 50 ml lotion base. Alternatively, use 20 drops for a warm compress (see p. 67).

For more recipes, see Chapter 14.

CHAPTER 14

Common Ailments and Conditions

*T*HE RECOMMENDATIONS in this chapter, for both physical and mental conditions, are for adult use; for the pregnant, young babies and children, see Chapters 12 and 13. Whilst I firmly believe that essential oils are often more effective than orthodox medication for minor ailments and conditions, readers should not endanger themselves or a member of their family by failing to consult a qualified medical practitioner in the event of a serious illness. The suggestions I offer are guidelines only, to help prevent disease, ease unnecessary suffering and support other treatments.

Because each person is different, I recommend several essential oils and usually alternative blends to try – and I hope you will experiment to find the oils that best suit your needs. When making your own blends, choose oils that complement each other (see Chapter 3, p. 42).

For methods of use (bath, compress, inhalant, etc.), see Chapter 6. Remember to use a 10 ml dropper bottle for measuring out drops.

Unless otherwise stated, proportions given for massage oils/lotions are for 50 ml base.

Measure guide • 1 ml = 30 drops approx.

Conditions and Treatments

ABSCESS ❦ BOIL

A localised collection of pus forming inflammation and swelling. If large it will need medical treatment.

Essential oils • Cajuput, camomile, lemon, lavender, tea-tree.

Formula for hot compress • 5 drops each of cajuput, lemon and thyme. Or, 5 drops each of camomile, lavender and tea-tree.

Apply the compress to the affected area twice a day, using up to a maximum 15 drops.

Tooth abscess • As a temporary measure, apply neat lavender or tea-tree with cotton-wool bud. Use an external compress (see p. 67). Seek a dentist's advice.

ACNE

Inflammation of the sebaceous glands of the skin, mainly in adolescents. Most commonly it forms on the face, but the chest and back can also be affected. (See also Chapter 12, pp. 160–61.)

Essential oils • Bergamot, cajuput, camomile (German or Roman), cedarwood, lavender, lemon, lemongrass, rose, sandalwood, tea-tree.

Formula • To 20 ml sweet almond or grapeseed oil, or bland lotion, add 4 drops each of bergamot, camomile, cedarwood.
Or, 4 drops lavender, 3 drops cajuput, 3 drops tea-tree, 2 drops lemongrass.

Apply to affected skin daily until improvement. Neat lavender or tea-tree may be applied directly to angry pustules.

Blemishes • To 20 ml base oil, add 6 drops rose, 6 drops sandalwood.
Apply daily until blemishes fade.

ANXIETY

A sense of uneasiness and agitation caused by apprehension or future misfortune; thoughts of impending doom. Excessive worry causing physical symptoms such as shaking, and/or feeling a tight knot or pain in the stomach.

Essential oils • Bergamot, camomile, clary sage, frankincense, lavender, lemon, rose, patchouli, petitgrain, sandalwood, thyme, vetiver. Basil and Spanish sage can be used, but sparingly.
To relieve tightness in the stomach area, massage the solar plexus region.
I believe an essence burner and an aromatic bath are the easiest and most effective self-help methods for treating anxiety. In the first four of the formulas below, blend

together the undiluted essential oils in a 10 ml dropper bottle. Use 6–10 drops in an essence burner and add 8–10 drops in a morning bath or shower two or three times a week.

Formula for working day • 4 ml grapefruit, 2 ml lavender, 2 ml lemon, 2 ml thyme.
Or, 5 ml bergamot, 5 ml frankincense.

Formula for rest-days or evening • 4 ml sandalwood, 4 ml ylang ylang, 2 ml clary sage.
Or, 4 ml camomile, 3 ml lavender, 3 ml patchouli or vetiver.

Blends to strengthen the nervous system • 5 ml basil, 5 ml bergamot. Or, 5 ml lemon and 5 ml Spanish sage or thyme.

Face oils or lotions • To 10 ml base, add 4 drops rose, 4 drops sandalwood, or, 4 drops petitgrain, 4 drops clary sage.

Body oils • Add 20–25 drops of one or more of the essential oils suggested above to 50 ml base. (If choosing basil or sage, use 5 drops once a week only.)

When you feel your treatment is working, try a maintenance programme, reducing treatment baths to once a week. Continue to use your essence burner regularly and have massage at least once a month.

ANGER

Feelings of rage or great annoyance – sometimes suppressed.

Essential oils • Camomile, frankincense, galbanum, lavender, peppermint, rose, ylang ylang.

Anger is best dealt with at the time – released, then calmed. If the anger is suppressed, it festers away causing untold problems. Try to explain how you feel rather than harbour a grudge, then perhaps any misunderstanding will be cleared up. If you cannot deal immediately with your anger, go where you can be alone and scream or, if at home, bash a pillow. Or, throw something (best if it is unbreakable but not so much fun or satisfaction). Forgive and let the anger go.

When dealing with suppressed anger, you might find some of the following oils helpful during any meditation or visualisation techniques you may be using.

To bring calm after the storm • blend 4 ml lavender, 2 ml camomile, 2 ml peppermint, 2 ml ylang ylang.
Or, 5 ml frankincense, 5 ml rose.

Use 6–10 drops in your essence burner or up to 10 drops in the bath. The last formula is expensive but worth every penny. If you cannot afford it, buy a pre-blended rose in jojoba oil, add 4–6 drops of frankincense, and use as a daily face oil.

Alternatively, massage the solar plexus.

ARTHRITIS

Inflammation of a joint or joints, characterised by pain and stiffness. *Osteoarthritis,* is a degenerative disease usually affecting older people. Wear-and-tear changes occur in the spine and the bones of the larger joints. *Rheumatoid arthritis* is a chronic disease of uncertain origin. It commonly starts in early adult life, especially in women, and emotional stress often appears to be a factor. The small joints of the fingers and toes are affected, causing swelling and intense pain.

Essential oils for osteoarthritis • Black pepper, cajuput, camomile, coriander, eucalyptus, juniper berry, lavender, lemon, marjoram, rose, rosemary. Also, Spanish sage (in moderation).

Massage formula • To 50 ml base, add 5 drops each of cajuput, coriander, lavender and lemon.
Or, 5 drops each of black pepper, camomile and rosemary, and 5 drops marjoram or rose.
Or, try any of the suggested essential oils singly, using 20 drops to 50 ml base oil.

For baths • Try the same blends as suggested for massage. Alternatively, use 3 drops each of cajuput, camomile, lavender and marjoram, or, 4 drops each of juniper berry, lemon and rosemary. You can use any of the suggested essential oils singly (up to 10 drops).

Essential oils for rheumatoid arthritis • As for osteoarthritis. Note, however, cajuput, camomile, lavender and rose are anti-inflammatory and particularly helpful.

Compress for inflamed, swollen joints • To 2 pints very cold water (use some ice cubes), add 5 drops each of cajuput and camomile and 5 drops lavender or rose.

ASTHMA

A respiratory condition in which the bronchial tubes become constricted, causing paroxysms of acute breathing difficulty. Increased secretion also tends to obstruct the air passages, causing wheezing. Asthma may be due to an allergy or be stress related. A predisposition to asthma is often inherited. The condition is often triggered by anxiety.

Aromatherapy may be used in conjunction with medical supervision.

Essential oils • Bergamot, cajuput, eucalyptus, lavender, lemon, niaouli, peppermint, pine, thyme. In moderation, i.e. half recommended amounts, hyssop and Spanish sage.

Formula • 3 ml each of eucalyptus, lavender, peppermint. Or, 3 ml each of bergamot, hyssop, lemon, niaouli.

This blend can be used in an essence burner (6–10 drops), or as an inhalant (4–5 drops). It is important to keep relaxed if you are asthmatic, so combine relaxing oils with your treatment. Consult an aromatherapist for regular treatment.

BLOOD-PRESSURE, HIGH

In medical terms, hypertension. The blood in the arterial system always circulates under pressure, but when this is too high problems can arise. Hypertension is sometimes associated with anxiety as well as medical conditions such as kidney diseases or glandular problems. Serious blood pressure conditions should be medically supervised.

Note. Do not use oil of rosemary if suffering from high blood pressure.

Essential oils to reduce high blood pressure • Cananga, clary sage, geranium, hyssop, lavender, melissa, rose, ylang ylang.

Regularly use any of the above oils in an essence burner, singly or in a blend (6–10 drops). Have warm relaxing baths and professional massage or aromatherapy.

Formula for bath/essence burner • 4 ml lavender or rose, 3 ml clary sage, 3 ml ylang ylang. Use up to 10 drops in a bath.

Massage formula • To 50 ml base add 5 drops each of melissa and ylang ylang and 5 drops lavender or rose.

BLOOD-PRESSURE, LOW

In medical terms, hypotension.

Essential oils to stimulate the blood pressure • Hyssop, rosemary.

To regulate the blood pressure, use 5 drops hyssop once or twice a week in a bath (or in an essence burner).

BOILS

See Abscess.

BRONCHITIS

Inflammation of the bronchial tubes. Symptoms are breathing difficulties and painful coughing.

Essential oils • Benzoin, bergamot, cajuput, cedarwood, cinnamon leaf, eucalyptus, galbanum, hyssop, lavender, myrrh, niaouli, peppermint, pine, sandalwood, Spanish sage, tea-tree, violet. For essence burner only: cinnamon leaf.

Before treating yourself or a member of your family, make sure it is not a medical emergency, as can happen in the very young or very old, or someone of an extremely nervous condition or weak constitution. There are lots of essential oils to choose from, and several methods to use.

Massage formula • To 50 ml base oil or lotion add 5 drops each of eucalyptus, hyssop, lavender and sandalwood.
Or, 8 drops each of cedarwood, niaouli and tea-tree.
Or, 5 drops each of bergamot, myrrh, peppermint and pine.
Apply to the chest, throat and back.

Formula for bath, burner or inhalation • 4 ml each of sandalwood and tea-tree, 2 ml pine or Spanish sage.

BRUISES

A discoloration of the skin due to blood escaping from the vessels in the underlying tissues that have become damaged. Some people bruise very easily owing to thin blood vessels.

Essential oils • Cajuput, lavender, tea-tree.

The most effective remedy for a bruise is arnica lotion, ointment or homoeopathic tablets, obtainable from health stores. The essential oils listed above are also excellent, easing initial pain and helping to bring out the bruise. Apply any of the suggested oils neat to the injury straight away, then follow with a compress (see p. 68).

If you bruise easily, to your regular bath add a blend of 5

drops cypress and 5 drops lavender or lemon. This helps strengthen blood vessels.

BURNS

A lesion of the tissue caused by excessive heat. Medically burns are classified in three degrees. First degree burns involve the skin and superficial tissues. Second and third degree burns involve the deeper tissues and bones. Treat only very minor first degree burns. For more serious burns seek medical advice.

Essential oils • Camomile, lavender, rose, rosemary, tea-tree.

The best first aid treatment is to apply neat lavender oil to the burn. You can put the burn under cold water first, but I have found that using neat lavender oil stops the pain very quickly and prevents blistering. If necessary, cover the burn with a sterile gauze and apply neat lavender at hourly intervals, or three times a day.

You can use the other oils listed by adding them to a cold water compress.

CATARRH

Inflammation of a mucous membrane associated with an excess secretion of mucus. Here we are concerned with catarrh affecting the nose and upper respiratory passages. If the catarrh is on the chest, see Bronchitis.

Essential oils • Basil, cedarwood, eucalyptus, fennel, frankincense, lavender, marjoram, myrrh, niaouli, peppermint, pine, sandalwood, tea-tree.

If you suffer from either acute or chronic catarrh, use one or a blend of these in an essence burner or as an inhalant on a regular basis until the condition improves. The following recipes are for essence burner (6–10 drops) or bath (up to 10 drops).

Formula for chronic catarrh • 3 ml basil, 3 ml marjoram, 2 ml cedarwood, 2 ml fennel.

Formula for acute catarrh • 4 ml each of eucalyptus and tea-tree, 2 ml niaouli.

CELLULITE

Fluids and toxins trapped in subcutaneous fat cells, causing a lumpy, puckered, orange-peel look to the skin, mainly on the thighs and hips. The condition appears to be connected with hormone balance, poor circulation or fluid retention.

Essential oils • Cypress, fennel, geranium, grapefruit, juniper berry, lavender, lemon, patchouli, rosemary.

Cellulite is notoriously difficult to get rid of. Diet is important. Aromatherapy, using detoxifying oils, has been found to be an effective form of treatment.

Massage formula 1 • To 50 ml base add 6 drops geranium, 6 drops juniper berry, 6 drops lemon, 4 drops fennel.

Massage formula 2 • 6 drops lavender, 6 drops patchouli, 6 drops rosemary, 4 drops cypress.

Using formula 1, massage affected areas every day for a month. Stop for four days, then change to formula 2 and start again. During the treatment period, add 6 drops of juniper berry to your bathwater twice a week and use a rough mit or brush on the affected areas. Drinking lots of still mineral water is supposed to help. Cut out unnecessary salt, sugar, fats, chocolates and red meat. Eat plenty of fibre-rich foods, green vegetables and fruit.

CIRCULATION, POOR

Sluggish blood flow in the tissues. Blood circulating around the body acts as a transport system for nutrients, oxygen and everything in the processes essential to maintain life. The blood is pumped by the heart which is divided into two halves. The right side collects spent, deoxygenated 'venous' blood from the body and pumps it to the lungs for re-oxygenation. The left side of the heart collects the revitalised blood from the lungs and pumps it with force through the arteries to the tissues of the body.

The major arteries and veins connect with smaller and smaller vessels, arterioles and venules. Eventually they become a network of microscopic vessels called capillaries which act as a connecting link between the arterioles and venules. If the circulation is poor, insufficient oxygen gets through to the tissues.

Essential oils • Bay, black pepper, coriander, ginger, juniper berry, lavender, marjoram, rose, rosemary, thyme.

Oils termed rubefacients (e.g. black pepper, rosemary) stimulate blood flow to localised areas. They cause the capillaries to widen, allowing a greater volume of blood and therefore extra oxygen to get through to the tissues.

The best method of improving general circulation is regular use of essential oils in massage or the bath. The first of the following recipes is a really spicy oil. If you have a sensitive skin, do a patch test first.

Massage oil • To 50 ml base add 6 drops rosemary, 5 drops bay, 5 drops coriander and 4 drops black pepper or ginger.

Or, 8 drops lavender, 6 drops rose and 6 drops rosemary or thyme.

For a bath • Use either of the above combinations, adjusting quantities, or a single oil, e.g. 10 drops rosemary.

COLD SORE

The medical name for cold sores is Herpes labialis. They are clusters of blisters that form on the outer rim of the lips caused by a viral infection.

Essential oils • Lavender, tea-tree.

Use a cotton bud and apply a little neat oil to the cold sore twice a day until clear.

COLDNESS, EMOTIONAL

Lack of feeling, inability to feel love or compassion.

Essential oils • Benzoin, lavender, melissa, rose, rosemary, ylang ylang.

Use pre-blended rose as a face oil or perfume. Alternatively, use 6–8 drops of rose in the bath.

If you cannot afford rose, try lavender, or a blend of 4 ml benzoin, 4 ml melissa, 2 ml ylang ylang. Add up to 10 drops in the bath or essence burner.

COLDS AND INFLUENZA

Colds are caused by virus infection of the upper respiratory tract, characterised by coughing and sneezing. There are some 30 different viruses, called rhinoviruses, that cause colds. There are others that cause influenza.

The symptoms of a cold are a running nose, 'thick' head and a general run-down feeling. Some people call a severe cold 'flu', and indeed a mild attack of influenza may resemble a cold. When the attack is sudden, with aching in the muscles of the limbs as well as fever, that is true influenza. Typically, the illness is followed by weakness, lack of vitality and sometimes depression. The more severe types of influenza, that sometimes come as epidemics, can be fatal. The greatest risk in these cases is secondary infection of the respiratory tract by bacteria, which is why antibiotics are prescribed by doctors.

Incidentally, antibiotics do not conflict with aromatherapy.

Seek medical advice if symptoms are severe.

Essential oils • Eucalyptus, lavender, lemon, pine, tea-tree, thyme.

The suggested oils may all be considered prophylactic, i.e. they help *prevent* the disease. At the first sign of a cold or influenza, have a comfortably hot aromatherapy bath –

Formula • 5 drops tea-tree, 5 drops lavender.
Or, 5 drops thyme, 5 drops lemon.

Use lavender, lemon, tea-tree or thyme in an essence burner (6–10 drops) or as a steam inhalation (4–5 drops), either singly or as a blend.

Dissolve a heaped teaspoon of honey in half a cup hot water and add the juice of a small lemon or half a large one. Drink three or four times a day. Also, take vitamin C tablets.

CONFIDENCE, LACK OF

Having no belief in one's abilities. No self-assurance.

Essential oils • Bergamot, cedarwood, frankincense, galbanum, geranium, jasmine, rose.

Most of us suffer to some extent from lack of confidence, and as a consequence we miss many of life's opportunities. I am not suggesting that merely by using essential oils a longstanding problem like this can be overcome. However, if you are studying for an exam or seeking ways to improve your confidence levels, aromatherapy can help.

I can recommend using pre-blended rose as a face oil or perfume. And try the following blend –

Formula • 3 ml basil, 3 ml cedarwood, 4 ml geranium.
Use 6–10 drops in an essence burner or 6–8 drops in a bath.

CONFUSION

A state of bewilderment or mental disorder; the mind lacks clarity.

Essential oils • Basil, cajuput, frankincense, grapefruit, rosemary, Spanish sage, tea-tree.

Confusion is not confined to the elderly – it can happen at any age. Usually it occurs through an inability to relax. When things get on top of you, a state of mild panic sets in causing confusion.

Formula for essence burner • 4 ml Spanish sage, 3 ml basil, 3 ml cajuput or tea-tree.

Use 6–10 drops, every day if needed.

Formula for bath • 5 drops frankincense, 5 drops grapefruit or rosemary.

Use two or three times a week.

Once you feel an improvement, maintain balance by using any of the suggested oils regularly in your essence burner or bath at least once a week.

CONSTIPATION

Sluggish action of bowels, which can affect any age group. If toxic matter is not released regularly, debility and depression result.

Essential oils • Black pepper, fennel, lavender, marjoram, orange, rosemary.

Massage oil/lotion • To 50 ml base add 5 drops each of black pepper, fennel, lavender, rosemary.

Massage the abdomen in a clockwise direction, to stimulate intestinal peristalsis (a muscular wave of contraction followed by relaxation). Do this twice a day for a week until regular movement is restored.

If the condition is persistent, consult an aromatherapist or reflexologist.

CRAMP

A very painful involuntary contraction of a muscle.

Essential oils • Cajuput, camomile, clary sage, ginger, lavender, lemon, marjoram, rosemary.

Cramp usually comes on during the night or early morning. If you are prone to cramp, a massage oil/lotion used every night may prevent attacks.

Massage formula • To 50 ml base add 5 drops each of cajuput, camomile, lavender and 5 drops black pepper or marjoram.

During an attack, rub the painful area with the oil/lotion. As soon as possible have a bath – a fairly hot one – adding 8 drops camomile and 8 drops lavender or marjoram. The combination of heat and oils will totally relax the muscles.

CUTS AND GRAZES

See First Aid.

CYSTITIS

Inflammation of the bladder, either acute or chronic. The symptoms are pain over the lower abdomen and urgency to pass water.

Essential oils • bergamot, eucalyptus, lavender, sandalwood.

Massage every day in conjunction with baths –

Massage oil • To 50 ml base add 10 drops sandalwood, 5 drops bergamot, 5 drops eucalyptus.

Formula for bath • 5 drops bergamot, 5 drops lavender.

For pain and irritation apply cold lavender-water compresses. Drink plenty of fluids such as diluted lemon juice, barley water or just plain water.

DEBILITY

Weakness, either physical (due to age or illness) or mental (after a breakdown or trauma).

Essential oils for physical debility • Clary sage, cypress, frankincense, ginger, lemon, rosemary, Spanish sage.

Essential oils for mental debility • Basil, bergamot, eucalyptus, lavender, peppermint, tea-tree, thyme.

Any kind of treatment for weakness should be gradual. Massage is an excellent way to regain strength, but start with only 15 minutes and then build up to at least an hour. The same applies to self-help reflexology – start with 10 minutes on each foot, increasing to 20 minutes.

Formula for physical debility • 4 ml cypress, 2 ml each of clary sage, frankincense, rosemary.

Add up to 10 drops in your bath. Relax for just 10 minutes. Take this bath twice a day if possible. The same formula can be used in a body oil.

Formula for mental debility • 3 ml basil, 3 ml eucalyptus, 2 ml bergamot, 2 ml tea-tree or thyme.

Use 6–10 drops in an essence burner or up to 10 drops in a bath until the condition improves.

Formula for mental and physical weakness • 3 ml clary sage, 3 ml frankincense, 2 ml basil or thyme, 2 ml bergamot or rosemary.

Use in essence burner or bath.

DEPRESSION

A low mental condition. It may range from a fed-up feeling to a severe medical condition, perhaps with a suicidal tendency. Despair, feelings of inadequacy, guilt, bereavement, worries, disturbed sleep, hormonal imbalance and illness can all lead to depression. Sometimes a person can be severely depressed without a known cause over a long period. In such a case medical help is required, and also whenever there is abnormal behaviour.

Aromatherapy can be a great help to the depressed. For post-natal depression, see pp. 153–54.

Essential oils • Bergamot, camomile, clary sage, frankincense, geranium, grapefruit, jasmine, lavender, lemongrass, melissa, neroli, orange, patchouli, rose, Spanish sage, sandalwood, ylang ylang.

Regular use of any of the suggested oils in an essence burner or bath will do much to alleviate feelings of gloom. The more expensive ones – jasmine, neroli and rose – can be bought pre-blended and used as a face oil or perfume. Have regular massage treatments.

Formula • 2 ml each of basil, bergamot, melissa, sandalwood, ylang ylang.
Or, 4 ml grapefruit, 3 ml clary sage, 3 ml geranium or jasmine.

Use 6–10 drops in an essence burner daily, or up to 10 drops in a bath two or three times a week.

Antidepressant face oil • To 20 ml base add 5 drops each of neroli, orange, petitgrain.

DERMATITIS

See Eczema.

DIARRHOEA

Loose and frequent evacuation of the bowels. Sometimes caused by a 'bug' or anxiety.

Essential oils • Camomile, ginger, lemon, neroli, peppermint, sandalwood.

If due to anxiety • To 25 ml base add 5 drops camomile, 5 drops peppermint, 5 drops sandalwood, 5 drops neroli or lavender.

Or, 10 drops peppermint, 10 drops camomile or sandalwood.

To avoid overstimulation of the intestines, apply the massage oil/lotion using very gentle movements. Alternatively, use the same combination of essential oils, or a single oil, in a compress. Drink camomile or peppermint herbal tea.

DYSPEPSIA

See Indigestion.

ECZEMA

Inflammation of the skin characterised by redness, itching, scaling, crusting and sometimes weeping. The condition appears to be associated with allergy and/or stress; sometimes there is a hereditary factor.

Essential oils • Bergamot, cajuput, camomile, cedarwood, geranium, juniper berry, lavender, patchouli, rose, sandalwood, tea-tree, ylang ylang.

When dealing with a dry eczema a massage oil will be helpful. For weepy eczema, try a bland lotion base or a compress.

Formula for dry eczema • To 50 ml base add 5 drops each of bergamot, geranium, sandalwood, 5 drops lavender or tea-tree.

Formula for weeping eczema • To 50 ml lotion add 10 drops patchouli, 5 drops juniper, 5 drops cedarwood or rose.

For a dry eczema bath, use lavender and ylang ylang (up to 10 drops in all).

EXHAUSTION

State of fatigue, weakness or collapse due to either physical or emotional causes – all the energies are used up.

Physical

Essential oils • Black pepper, frankincense, ginger, grapefruit, rosemary.

Formula • 4 ml frankincense, 3 ml grapefruit, 3 ml ginger or rosemary.

The blend may be used in a massage oil, or in a bath (up to 10 drops). Alternatively, for a bath, use 10 drops of black pepper.

Mental

Essential oils • Basil, lemongrass, rosemary, thyme.

Formula • 4 ml basil, 3 ml lemongrass, 3 ml thyme.
Use 6–10 drops in an essence burner or up to 10 drops in a bath.

General tiredness, including jet lag

Essential oils • Frankincense, grapefruit, rosemary.

Formula • To 50 ml base add 8 drops grapefruit, 6 drops frankincense, 6 drops rosemary.

Use up to 10 drops in the bath.

FIBROSITIS

Inflammation of fibrous tissue of muscle sheaths.

Essential oils • Cajuput, camomile, lavender, lemon, rose, rosemary, tea-tree.

Massage oil/lotion • To 50 ml base add 5 drops each of cajuput, camomile, rosemary, 5 drops lavender or lemon.

The areas most prone to fibrositis are the shoulders – very difficult to treat yourself. Ask your partner to massage them, or have professional remedial massage. Alternatively, soak in a fairly hot aromatic bath.

Formula for bath • 4 drops camomile, 3 drops cajuput, 3 drops lavender.

FIRST AID

For serious accidents, seek medical attention.

Bruises • Apply neat lavender oil (see p. 179).

Burns • Apply neat lavender or tea-tree oil (see p. 180).

Cuts, grazes • Apply neat lavender oil. If necessary, cover with a plaster. You will be amazed and delighted to see how quickly wounds heal using this method.

Fainting • Inhale Spanish sage or tea-tree oil, either direct from the bottle or on a tissue or pad.

Insect bites, stings • Apply neat lavender, lemon or tea-tree oil. Pull sting out with tweezers if visible.

Shock, panic, hysteria • Inhale marjoram, melissa, rose or tea-tree oil, under the nose, either in a bottle or on a pad. Also use an essence burner with 6–8 drops of marjoram.

FLUID RETENTION (OEDEMA)

An excess of fluid in the tissues, causing distension and swelling, which may be either localised or affect the whole body. It can come about for a number of different reasons. One of the most common is premenstrual tension (see p. 208). In pregnancy there is often fluid retention though this is usually quite normal (a protection for the foetus) and nothing to worry about. Localised, temporary swelling occurs in injuries such as a sprains. Puffy ankles can come about from standing for long periods (see p. 149). Fluid trapped in the fatty tissues is associated with cellulite (see p. 181). More generalised fluid retention is often associated with overweight, though it can indicate serious illness, such as kidney, liver or heart disease, which should be under medical supervision.

Diuretics (e.g. fennel, juniper berry) increase the flow of urine, which can help in fluid retention. They should only be used for short periods and not at all in kidney disease.

Generalised fluid retention

Essential oils • Fennel, geranium, grapefruit, juniper berry, lavender, lemon, parsely (in moderation), patchouli, Spanish sage.

Massage oil • To 50 ml base add 5 drops each of fennel, lemon, patchouli, 5 drops juniper berry or lavender.
Or, 10 drops lemon, 5 drops grapefruit, 5 drops lavender.

Any of the above recipes can be used in a bath two or three times a week, adjusting the drops up to 10.

FOOT CONDITIONS

Proper care of the feet affects one's general well-being and comfort.

Excessive odour/sweating • Regular footbaths will combat this. Add up to 10 drops cypress to a bowl of warm water, soak the feet for 15 minutes and dry thoroughly.

For a massage lotion, to 50 ml base add 20 drops cypress, 5 drops lemon or peppermint.

Verrucas (warts) • Apply neat lavender, lemon or tea-tree oil to each verruca three times a day until the condition improves.

Tired feet • Have a foot bath as above but with 5 drops each of eucalyptus and peppermint.

GLANDULAR FEVER

An acute viral disease, mildly contageous; symptoms are swelling of the lymph glands, sore throat, fever and malaise. Medical treatment is required but aromatherapy given in conjunction with it can boost the immune system and aid recovery. The illness can drag on for weeks, with the patient becoming very debilitated and depressed. Massage is not recommended during the acute stage.

Essential oils • Frankincense, lavender, rosemary, tea-tree, thyme.

Massage lotion/compress for glands • 10 drops frankincense, 5 drops lavender, 5 drops thyme.
Or, 10 drops bergamot, 10 drops tea-tree.

Apply the lotion very gently or apply a compress to the areas affected.

Formula for bath • 3 drops each of frankincense, tea-tree, thyme.

Initially take this bath every other day for 2–3 weeks. Then maintain the routine two or three times a week until improvement is felt. If feeling very tired, alternate 3 drops of rosemary with tea-tree. Regular massage and reflexology will help recovery during convalescence.

GOUT

Inflammation and swelling of the hands and feet associated with excessive uric acid levels in the blood.

Essential oils • Cajuput, camomile, juniper berry, lavender, lemon, marjoram, rose.

Massage oil • To 50 ml base add 10 drops lemon, 5 drops cajuput, 5 drops marjoram.
Or, 5 drops juniper berry, 5 drops lavender, 10 drops camomile or rose.

If there is considerable pain or inflammation, the above formula can also be used in a cold compress (15 drops) or foot-bath (10 drops).

Buy pre-blended rose, which can be used on its own or blended with the other oils. Apply to the affected area once or twice a day.

GRIEF ❦ ANGUISH

Misery, intense pain of an emotional or mental nature due to, for example, bereavement, loss of a pet or divorce.

Essential oils • Camomile, cypress, jasmine, lavender, marjoram, rose, vetiver.

The above oils will be found comforting. Sniff them in the bottle like smelling salts. After the initial shock, use the oils regularly, either singly or in combination.

Formula • 4 ml camomile, 3 ml lavender, 3 ml marjoram.

Use 6–10 drops in your essence burner, up to 10 drops in a bath or 3–4 drops on your pillow at night. Continue treatment for as long as required.

Face oil • To 10 ml base oil/lotion, add 8 drops of rose or jasmine, or 4 drops of each.

Initially use every day, then once or twice a week.

GUILT

Self-reproach. A feeling of having done something wrong or failed to do something that should have been done – happens all the time amongst families!

Essential oils • Lavender, myrrh, pine, rose, sandalwood, ylang ylang.

Guilt can be a very destructive emotion. The above oils are a valuable adjunct either to self-help or psychotherapy.

Formula • 3 ml lavender, 3 ml pine, 4 ml myrrh or ylang ylang.

Use 6–10 drops in an essence burner or up to 10 drops in a bath.

HAEMORRHOIDS (PILES)

Swollen, protruding veins in the region of the anus and lower rectum, often painful and bleeding.

Essential oils • Cypress, lavender, lemon.

The most effective method of treating this complaint is to use a bidet or bath.

Bidet formula • 3 drops cypress, 3 drops lemon.

Swish the water well to disperse the oil. If your skin is very sensitive, add 1 treaspoon of almond oil or milk. Sit for 5-10 minutes. Repeat several times a day if possible.

Soothing lotion • To 50 ml bland lotion add 10 drops cypress, 5 drops lavender, 5 drops lemon.

Apply twice a day. At night, soak a soft ball of cotton wool in the lotion and place on the affected area (wear protective pants to keep the swab in place).

HALITOSIS

Bad breath, generally caused by digestive problems, bad teeth or smoking.

Essential oils • Bergamot, fennel, lavender, myrrh, peppermint, tea-tree, thyme.

Mouthwash (ready-to-use) • To 100 ml water in a bottle add 3 drops bergamot, 3 drops lavender, 3 drops peppermint, 3 drops tea-tree or thyme and (optional) a teaspoon of cheap brandy or vodka. Shake well and use immediately. Make sure you do not swallow.

Mouthwash concentrate • 5 ml cheap brandy or vodka, 5 ml each of bergamot, fennel, lavender, peppermint and 5 ml tea-tree or thyme. Shake well in a bottle and use 4–5 drops in half a tumbler of warm water once or twice a day.

HEADACHE

Pain in the head usually caused by dilation of the cerebral arteries, muscle contraction or insufficient oxygen. Sinus infection (p. 216) and catarrh (p. 180) can also cause headaches.

Headaches that are persistent and severe, or have no apparent cause, are a possible sign of a more serious disorder; seek medical advice.

For Migraine, see p. 209.

Essential oils • Basil, cajuput, eucalyptus, lavender, lemon, marjoram, peppermint, rose, rosemary.

Formula • 4 ml peppermint, 3 ml rosemary, 3 ml basil or lemon.
Or, 4 ml lavender, 3 ml eucalyptus, 3 ml cajuput or marjoram.

Use 6–10 drops in an essence burner or up to 10 drops in a bath. Alternatively, put a few drops on a cotton pad and inhale. Try a few drops on the pillow at night.

INDECISION

Inability to make up one's mind about specific issues ranging from moving house to what to wear, causing unnecessary tension. It comes from a fear of being wrong or appearing so to others. Learn to make firm, positive decisions in your life and to trust your intuition. You will then find the problem disappears.

Essential oils • Basil, bergamot, cardamom, cypress, galbanum, grapefruit, myrrh, rosemary.

The above oils, used in combination or singly, can help you develop the capacity for positive, decisive action.

Formula • 3 ml each of basil, bergamot, cardamom.
Or, 3 ml cypress, 3 ml myrrh, 3 ml grapefruit or rosemary.

Use 6–10 drops in an essence burner regularly. If you have an important decision to make, relax in a bath with up to 10 drops of the same formula or any one of the suggested oils. Meditate and the answer will come.

INDIGESTION

Difficulty in digesting food, with pain, heartburn and belching. Food that is too fatty may cause indigestion. Sometimes it is due to tension and anxiety. To avoid ulcers, relax whilst eating.

Essential oils • Camomile, cardamom, fennel, ginger, peppermint or spearmint.

Massage oil • To 20 ml base add 6 drops camomile, 6 drops ginger or peppermint.
Or, 6 drops cardamom, 6 drops fennel, 4 drops peppermint.

If you continually suffer from indigestion, regularly massage the stomach region with any of the above blends and drink fennel or peppermint tea.

For instant relief, add 2 drops peppermint oil to a cup of boiled water and sip slowly.

INSOMNIA

Sleeplessness. Difficulty in falling asleep and/or failing to achieve uninterrupted sleep can be a temporary or a longstanding problem. Try hypnotherapy or acupuncture if aromatherapy does not help.

Essential oils • Basil, camomile, clary sage, lavender, marjoram, neroli, orange, rose, sandalwood, ylang ylang.

Formula • 4 ml orange, 3 ml lavender, 3 ml sandalwood.
Or, 3 ml basil, 3 ml marjoram, 4 ml camomile, neroli or rose.

You might prefer to experiment with different combinations. For example, a blend of equal parts of bergamot and ylang ylang is often effective.

Two hours prior to bedtime • Use 6–10 drops of one of the suggested blends in your essence burner.

One hour before retiring • Have a warm bath with either 4 drops clary sage or up to 10 drops lavender.

Try 3–4 drops of lavender or ylang ylang on your pillow, or neroli or rose face oil. One of my clients drank a wineglass of lettuce juice before bed and found it most effective.

Too much TV can disturb sleep. Resist tea, coffee or 'coke' during the evening – have a cup of herb tea instead.

IRRITABILITY

Over-sensitivity, with difficulty controlling annoyance or anger – being snappy.

Essential oils • Camomile, lavender, lemon, mandarin, melissa, rose, rosewood.

Formula • 4 ml lavender, 3 ml mandarin, 3 ml camomile or rose.
Or, 3 ml each of melissa, marjoram and rosewood.

Use 6–10 drops in an essence burner or up to 10 drops in a bath. Have regular massage if possible. Also, try to find an explanation for irritability (dissatisfaction with your life, overwork, PMT), and look for ways to change things.

JEALOUSY

When you wish that you could have something someone else has. Jealousy is a destructive emotion and occasionally so strong it leads to murder. It can also become obsessive.

Essential oil • Jasmine, lavender, rose, ylang ylang.

Rose, in my opinion, is the best oil to help jealousy, but if it is unobtainable use any of the other oils. If the problem is obsessive, seek qualified advice. Have massage and reflexology to help balance the emotions and promote self-esteem.

KIDNEY CONDITIONS

The kidneys extract surplus water from the bloodstream, regulate the concentration of salts in the blood and excrete waste products. They also regulate blood pressure. These are all vital processes, so for any kidney condition, such as infections or stones, it is absolutely essential to get prompt medical aid. Some essential oils are kidney tonics, enhancing the filtration of the kidneys.

Essential oils (kidney tonics) • Clary sage, juniper, lavender.

Kidney tonic massage formula • To 50 ml base add 10 drops lavender, 10 drops clary sage or juniper.

Massage back and front between hip bone and lower chest. Use up to 10 drops of the blend or any one of the suggested oils in the bath.

LARYNGITIS

Inflammation of the larynx, frequently accompanied by cough, hoarseness or loss of voice, and dry sore throat.

Essential oils • Benzoin, bergamot, cajuput, Spanish sage, sandalwood, thyme.

Massage formula • To 50 ml base add 10 drops cajuput, 5 drops sage, 5 drops thyme.
Or, 10 drops bergamot.

Massage the throat and neck area, from the chin to the breastbone. Do this twice a day until improvement is felt. Also try a gargle with 1 teaspoon of honey and 4 drops of cajuput in a cup of warm water.

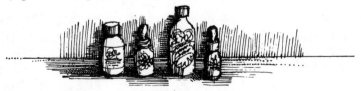

LETHARGY

A state of lassitude and lack of energy which may be due to a physical condition such as illness, or from a state of mind. If it is the latter and it is serious, counselling may be necessary. But generally a good stimulating massage will do the trick.

Essential oils • Cajuput, eucalyptus, ginger, lemongrass, peppermint, rosemary.

Formula • 4 ml ginger, 3 ml eucalyptus, 3 ml peppermint. Or, 4 ml lemograss, 4 ml rosemary, 3 ml cajuput.

Regularly use 6–10 drops in an essence burner and up to 10 drops in a bath. After your bath, give your body a very brisk rub with a skin brush or bath mit. This will stimulate the blood flow and pep up the system.

LIVER CONDITIONS

The liver is the largest gland in the body and is situated in the upper right part of the abdominal cavity, immediately below the diaphragm. It secretes bile, detoxifies poisons and has several other important functions. Serious liver diseases must be medically supervised. However, at times we all feel liverish, perhaps through too much indulgence in alcohol or rich, fatty foods. A number of essential oils stimulate liver function in different ways, such as easing congestion and acting as a tonic.

Essential oils • Camomile, fennel, juniper, lemon, peppermint, rose, rosemary.

Liver congestion massage formula • To 50 ml base add 6 drops each of camomile, fennel, peppermint.

Liver tonic • 8 drops lemon, 6 drops juniper, 6 drops rose or rosemary.

To improve liver function, massage the liver area with the tonic oil every day for two weeks. Drink camomile or peppermint herbal tea and, every morning, a tablespoonful of fresh lemon juice diluted in warm water. Dandelion coffee is also a good liver tonic.

LONELINESS

A feeling of unhappiness through isolation or not having anyone to communicate with.

Loneliness can be felt even in a crowded room, if you are unable join in or feel part of the group. Elderly people sometimes feel abandoned, which can be very distressing. Counselling and aromatherapy may help to relieve the problem.

Use marjoram and/or rose in a essence burner (6–10 drops), or in a bath (up to 10 drops). Or use rose in a face oil or perfume.

LUMBAGO

Pain in the low back involving muscles and ligaments.

Essential oils • Black pepper, cajuput, camomile, ginger, lavender, lemon, niaouli, rosemary.

It is important to rest and keep the lower back warm. Aromatherapy massage and baths will alleviate the discomfort.

Massage oil • To 50 ml base add 8 drops each of black pepper, cajuput and lavender.
Or, 8 drops each of camomile, ginger and lemon.

Apply twice a day.

For bath • Up to 10 drops niaouli or rosemary, or 5 drops of each.
Or, 5 drops each of camomile and lavender.

MEMORY, POOR

Slow recall, often due to mental fatigue and/or poor concentration, or senility.

The mind should be looked after as well as the body. Crossword puzzles are an excellent way to keep your mind in trim.

Essential oils • Basil, rosemary, thyme.

Formula • 4 ml rosemary, 3 ml basil, 3 ml thyme.

Use 6–10 drops regularly in an essence burner.

MENOPAUSE PROBLEMS

The menopause is the cessation of menstruation. It occurs at a time in a woman's life termed the climacteric or change of life. Usually the process takes place over a year or two and between the ages of 43 and 55. The ovaries at this time cease to produce eggs and the body goes through hormonal changes, particularly oestrogen loss. Although the change of life is a normal process through which all women pass, many will experience quite distressing side effects, such as hot flushes, mood swings, palpitations and insomnia.

By having regular aromatherapy treatments and reflexology, women from the age of 42 onward may well avert some of these unwanted symptoms.

Essential oils • Camomile, clary sage, cypress, fennel, geranium, jasmine, lavender, neroli, rose, Spanish sage, sandalwood.

Massage formula • To 50 ml base add 5 drops each of clary sage, cypress, fennel and lavender.

Massage the lower abdomen (ovary area) two or three times a week. Also have geranium baths (8 drops) once or twice a week.

Face oil • To 20 ml base oil/lotion add 4 drops each of jasmine, rose and sandalwood.
Or, 4 drops each of camomile, geranium, lavender.

Use face oil two or three times a week. Pre-blended neroli could also be used.

Massage lotion for hot flushes/night sweats • To 50 ml base add 10 drops cypress, 10 drops Spanish sage.

Massage your feet with the lotion every night before going to bed. Avoid alcohol and spicy foods, drink lots of chilled still mineral water and take vitamin C tablets.

Formula for depression/mood swings • 4 ml geranium, 3 ml clary sage, 3 ml lavender.
Or, 10 ml neroli or petitgrain.

Regularly use 6–10 drops in an essence burner or up to 10 drops in the bath. If the depression is severe, try a camomile and lavender bath (5 drops of each) twice a week. The massage oil recommended for hot flushes is also helpful for depression. Massage over the ovary area.

MENSTRUATION PROBLEMS

Some of the problems that can occur are: *amenorrhoea,* the abnormal absence of the period; *dysmenorrhoea,* period pain; *menorrhagia,* excessive bleeding. The periods may also be scanty and/or irregular.

The massage oils/lotions suggested below for specific problems should be used once or twice a day for 10 days prior to your period (50 ml base).

Absence of period • 5 drops each clary sage, fennel, rose and rosemary.

Painful periods • 10 drops cajuput, 10 drops camomile, 5 drops peppermint. (Also use during the period.)

Excessive bleeding • 10 drops frankincense, 8 drops cypress, 8 drops lemon.

Irregular periods • 10 drops clary sage, 10 drops cypress, 5 drops fennel.

Scanty periods • 5 drops each of camomile, lavender, rose and rosemary.

PMT• 5 drops camomile, 10 drops cypress, 10 drops lavender.

MIGRAINE

Recurrent, usually one-sided headache. It may be accompanied by disturbance of vision, nausea, vomiting and prostration.

Essential oils • Cajuput, camomile, eucalyptus, lavender, lemon, marjoram, melissa, peppermint, rosemary.

Formula • 4 ml lemon, 3 ml cajuput, 3 ml lavender or melissa.

Use 6–10 drops of the blend, or any of the oils suggested, in an essence burner, and up to 10 drops in a bath. Alternatively, put a few drops on a cotton pad and inhale, or a few drops on your pillow.

MOUTH ULCERS

A sore on the mucus membrane of the mouth, often occurring when a person is a little run down in health.

Essential oils • Myrrh, tea-tree, thyme.

Apply a little neat tea-tree oil directly using a cotton bud. Blot the area before swallowing.

Mouthwash • To a glass of warm water add 2 drops myrrh, 2 drops thyme.

Use twice a day.

MUSCULAR AILMENTS

The skeletal muscles are subject to damage or malfunction due to injury, overwork, stress and strain. If you over-exercise, the muscles are deprived of oxygenated blood, thereby weakening the fibres and rendering them vulnerable to injury. See also Rheumatism.

Essential oils • Black pepper, cajuput, camomile, clary sage, coriander, eucalyptus, ginger, juniper, lavender, lemon, lemongrass, marjoram, pine, rosemary.

Massage benefits muscles, keeping them free from toxicity and increasing the amount of oxygenated blood to the fibres.

General aches and pains • To 50 ml base, add 5 drops each of cajuput, eucalyptus, ginger, lavender.
Or, 5 drops each of juniper, lemon, rosemary, and 5 drops of black pepper or camomile.

Use twice a day for two weeks until improvement is obtained. Then maintain by using two or three times a week, alternating with the bath formula below.

Slack tone • 10 drops rosemary, 5 drops black pepper, 5 drops lemongrass or lemon.

Spasm/cramp • 5 drops each of cajuput, camomile, lavender, marjoram.

General stiffness • 5 drops each of coriander, ginger, juniper, lemon.

Bath formula • 4 drops rosemary, 3 drops camomile, 3 drops marjoram or pine.
Or, 4 drops lavender, 3 drops clary sage, 3 drops coriander.

An aromatherapy bath can help relax tired, overworked muscles.

NAUSEA

A feeling of sickness without actually vomiting.

Essential oils • Black pepper, fennel, peppermint.

Massage formula • To 50 ml base add 10 drops of peppermint, 5 drops black pepper, 5 drops fennel.

Massage the stomach area twice a day. Use peppermint oil in an essence burner and drink fennel or peppermint herbal tea. For Morning Sickness see p. 146.

NEGATIVITY

Lacking positive energies or qualities; little or no enthusiam for life; always expecting the worst; hypochondria. See also Anxiety.

Essential oils • Basil, bergamot, clary sage, frankincense, geranium, jasmine, lemon, lemongrass, myrrh, sandalwood.

Formula • 4 ml sandalwood, 3 ml bergamot, 3 ml clary sage or frankincense.
Or, 3 ml clary sage, 3 ml lemongrass, 3 ml geranium or jasmine.

Regularly use 6–10 drops in an essence burner or up to 10 drops in the bath.

NERVOUS TENSION

Too much stress on the nervous system, causing sufferers to be excitable, jumpy or irritable. Mostly affects the highly strung.

Essential oils (calming to the nerves) • Benzoin, bergamot, camomile, cedarwood, clary sage, geranium, jasmine, lavender, mandarin, marjoram, neroli, patchouli, rose, rosewood, sandalwood, ylang ylang.

Essential oils (nerve-strengthening) • Basil, bergamot, frankincense, lemon, Spanish sage, thyme.

The best plan is to make a calming formula and add one of the strengthening oils.

Massage formula • To 50 ml base add 5 drops each of mandarin, sandalwood and ylang ylang and 5 drops frankincense.

Formula for bath/essence burner • 3 ml bergamot, 3 ml lavender, 2 ml geranium, 2 ml basil or Spanish sage.

Use up to 10 drops in the bath and 6–10 drops in your essence burner.

OEDEMA

See Fluid Retention

PALPITATIONS

Rapid, forceful beating of the heart of which the person is aware. If persistent, it may be a sign of high blood pressure or a heart problem. Palpitations can also be a side effect of the change of life, or caused by anxiety. If the condition continues and is accompanied by pain or light-headedness, seek medical help.

Essential oils • Lavender, melissa, rose, ylang ylang.

Massage formula • To 50 ml base add 8 drops lavender, 8 drops ylang ylang, 4 drops melissa or rose.

Apply to heart and solar plexus areas.

Formula for bath • 5 drops each of lavender, melissa, ylang ylang.

PANIC ATTACK

Being overwhelmed with terror for no apparent reason. The condition can come on at any time, often with gasping, rapid breathing.

Essential oils • Basil, clary sage, frankincense, lavender, rose, tea-tree, vetiver.

Formula for preventing attacks • To 50 ml base add 10 drops frankincense, 10 drops lavender or rose.
Or, add a few drops clary sage to pre-blended rose oil.

At onset of an attack • Waft a bottle of frankincense, lavender or tea-tree under the nose like smelling salts. Do not inhale too deeply, however, as you may feel dizzy.

   In addition to aromatherapy treatment, massage the solar plexus area.

PHLEBITIS

Inflammation of a vein, usually affecting a leg. Characteristic symptoms are swelling, pain and tenderness. The leg looks white and feels heavy.

Essential oils • Camomile, lavender, lemon.

Phlebitis should not be massaged. Make a cold compress using the above oils, or add them to a warm bath.

PREMENSTRUAL TENSION (PMT)

See p. 208.

PSORIASIS

A non-infective chronic skin disease characterised by dry, scaly, red areas, most commonly in the flexure area of elbows, knees and wrists.

The cause is unknown, though worry and stress are predisposing factors. Aromatherapy treatment of this intractable condition is mainly aimed at quelling anxiety and stress and stimulating the growth of new skin cells to replace the damaged ones.

Essential oils • Bergamot, cajuput, camomile, cedarwood, geranium, lavender, rose, rosewood, sandalwood.

Lotion • To 50 ml base, add 8 drops each of bergamot, cajuput and geranium.
Or, 5 drops each of camomile, lavender, sandalwood, 5 drops cedarwood or rose.

Apply twice a day until there is an improvement, then once a day. Maintain improvement using the lotion twice a week. If the condition flares up again, increase the application until it subsides. Try different combinations if no marked improvement is seen.

Also add a few drops of lavender or sandalwood to your bath.

RHEUMATISM

In medical terminology, rheumatism embraces a whole range of disorders involving painful muscles and joints, including rheumatoid arthritis and osteoarthritis. In general usage, however, rheumatism is confined to conditions where the pain is mainly in the muscles rather than the joint itself. This is the kind of rheumatism that principally concerns us here. It often occurs after getting getting cold and wet, in damp weather, from being in a draught, etc.

Aromatherapy treatment concentrates on eliminating toxins, stimulating the circulation, and easing pain and muscle stiffness.

Essential oils • Black pepper, cajuput, camomile, eucalyptus, lavender, lemon, marjoram, rosemary, Spanish sage, thyme.

Massage formula • To 50 ml base add 8 drops lemon, 8 drops rosemary, 8 drops cajuput or eucalyptus.
Or, 8 drops camomile, 8 drops lavender, 8 drops marjoram or Spanish sage.

To ease rheumatism, it is a good idea to have regular massage. Also use the above combinations or any of the suggested oils in a bath (up to 10 drops).

SEXUAL RESPONSE, LOW

The problem is usually psychological and may need professional help. Anxiety is a frequent cause of frigidity or impotence. Physical disorders, such as diabetes, affect sexual response (seek medical advice).

Essential oils • Cedarwood, clary sage, fennel, jasmine, rosemary, sandalwood, ylang ylang.

To arouse sexual response in your partner, massage the erogenous zones with light, stroking movements using a blend of essential oils reputed to be aphrodisiacs. If impotence or frigidity does not respond, seek qualified counselling.

Lovers' blend • To 30 ml base add 5 drops sandalwood, 5 drops ylang ylang, 3 drops fennel, 2 drops clary sage.

SINUSITIS

Inflammation of an air sinus – a bony cavity in the skull. There is one on each side of the nose (the maxillary sinuses), and two at the root of the nose in the frontal bone (the frontal sinuses). Like the nose, they are lined with mucuous membrane.

The symptoms of sinusitis include pain in the forehead or around the eyes, nasal congestion and headache. Acute sinusitis may follow a cold and the patient suffers from a severe headache – prompt medical supervision should be sought. In chronic sinusitis the pain is duller, and there is constant mucus discharge in the nose that may be caused by allergy.

Essential oils • Cedarwood, lemon, eucalyptus, geranium, hyssop, lavender, niaouli, peppermint, pine.

Formula • 3 ml cedarwood, 3 ml lemon, 2 ml hyssop, 2 ml lavender.
Or, 3 ml geranium, 3 ml niaouli, 2 ml eucalyptus, 2 ml peppermint.

Either of the above combinations can be used in steam inhalation (see p. 69). To prevent sinusitis, use any of the suggested oils or blends in your essence burner.

SORE THROAT

Soreness and swelling of the throat due to infection (colds, flu), smoking or a dusty atmosphere.

Essential oils • Bergamot, cajuput, lavender, lemon, geranium, tea-tree, thyme.

The same essential oils are recommended for tonsilitis.

Massage formula for throat area • To 50 ml base add 8 drops each of bergamot, lavender, tea-tree or thyme.

Gargle • To a cup of warm water add 1 teaspoon honey and 2 drops each of lavender, lemon, tea-tree. Stir well, gargle in the usual way (do not swallow).

SPRAINS

See p. 68.

STRESS AND STRAIN

Over-exertion, mental and physical, where all the resources are taxed.

Essential oils • Basil, bergamot, frankincense, neroli, ylang ylang.

Relaxation is not the only requirement in this situation. Learn how to avoid taking on too much!

Formula • 3 ml bergamot, 3 ml frankincense, 2 ml basil, 2 ml neroli or ylang ylang.

Regularly use 6–10 drops in an essence burner or up to 10 drops in a bath. Have regular massage.

SUNBURN

Sore red patches on the skin as a result of having spent too much time in the hot sunshine. Fair skinned people are particularly susceptible.

Essential oils • Bergamot, camomile, lavender, sandalwood.

In the event of sunburn, apply neat lavender to the affected part. This will ease pain and prevent blistering.

Do not use bergamot just prior or during sunbathing as it is one of the oils that are classed as phototoxic. It is safe to use afterwards, however, and is effective used in an after-sun oil or lotion.

After-sun soothing oil/lotion • To 50 ml base, add 6 drops bergamot, 6 drops lavender, 5 drops camomile, 5 drops sandalwood.

TEARFULNESS

Proneness to tears for no apparent reason, though often linked with PMT and the menopause.

Essential oils • Cypress, geranium, lavender, marjoram, neroli.

Formula • 3 ml lavender, 3 ml marjoram, 2 ml cypress, 2 ml neroli or geranium.

Use 6–10 drops in an essence burner or up to 10 drops in a bath. A neroli face oil at night or used as a perfume will also help.

TONSILITIS

Inflammation of the tonsils, lymphoid tissue at the back of the throat.

Treatment is as recommended for Sore Throat.

THRUSH

Infection of mucus membrane by the fungus Candida albicans. The vagina is most commonly affected.

Essential oils • Lemon, tea-tree.

Formula for vaginal swab • To a cup of warm water add 2 drops each of lemon and tea-tree oil.

With a cotton wool pad, swab just inside the vagina. Alternatively, use the same formula to bathe the affected area in a bidet, using 4–5 drops and swishing the water well.

Plain live yoghurt is a well known and successful remedy for thrush. Eat the yoghurt on an empty stomach so its assimilation is fast. The yoghurt may also be used on a swab. A good method is to soak a tampon or cotton wool ball in a teaspoon of yoghurt plus 2 drops of tea-tree oil. Put the tampon just inside the vagina before going to bed and leave it overnight.

Ready made tea-tree cream can be purchased. Keep it in the fridge so that it is nice and cold on application to the vagina.

TOOTHACHE

Pain, either dull or acute, from a decayed tooth, often radiating to the face.

Essential oils • Clove, lavender, tea-tree.

To relieve the pain before getting to a dentist, use a small amount of any of the above oils neat on the painful tooth.

VARICOSE VEINS

Dilated veins, in particular in the legs, due to loss of elasticity in the vessel walls and valves so that the blood flow becomes inefficient. The condition causes aching and tiredness in the limbs. Ulceration can occur.

Essential oils • Cypress, lemon.

Never massage below the varicosity, as this will cause more swelling of the vein. Light, upward strokes from the affected area are helpful, however. Do not massage too deeply.

Lotion • To 50 ml base add 10 drops cypress, 10 drops lemon.

Lightly stroke the affected area twice a day. Whenever possible the limbs should be rested in an elevated position (above waist level).

For varicose ulcers • Use 15–20 drops tea-tree in a cold compress. Add the same number of drops to 50 ml base for an oil or lotion.

Pure honey is also a good healing agent. Apply the purest honey to the ulcer and cover with a lint dressing. Change and reapply dressings frequently. Drink plenty of camomile tea to aid healing.

WRINKLES

Creasing of the skin as it gets older, particularly noticeable on the face. The wrinkling is caused by the underlying support, i.e. collagen connective tissue, diminishing.

Essential oils • Frankincense, lemon.

Massage oil/lotion • To 50 ml base add 15 drops lemon, 10 drops frankincense.

When using the oil or lotion on the face, avoid the delicate eye area. Use regularly, at least once or twice a week.

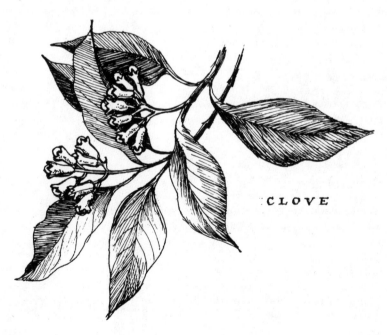

CLOVE

Suggested Reading

Aromatherapy

Patricia Davis, *Aromatherapy: an A–Z*, C.W. Daniel & Co., 1988.
Marcel Lavabre, *Aromatherapy Workbook*, Healing Arts Press, Vermont, 1990.
Julia Lawless, *The Encyclopaedia of Essential Oils*, Element Books, 1992.
Daniäle Ryman, *The Encyclopaedia of Plant Oils and How They Help You*, Piatkus Books, 1991.
Wanda Sellar, *The Directory of Essential Oils*, C.W. Daniel & Co., 1992.
Valerie Ann Worwood, *The Fragrant Pharmacy*, MacMillan, 1990.

Massage

Nigel Dawes & Fiona Harrold, *Massage Cures*, Thorsons, 1990.
Clare Maxwell-Hudson, *The Complete Book of Massage*, Dorling Kindersley.

Reflexology

Ann Gillanders, *Reflexology: The Ancient Answer to Modern Ailments*, Jenny Lee Publishing, 1987.

Self Growth

Louise L. Hay, *The Power is Within You*, Eden Grove Editions, 1991.

Louise L. Hay, *You Can Heal Your Life,* Eden Grove Editions, 1984.

Florence Scovell Shinn, *The Game of Life and How to Play It,* 39th edition, L.N. Fowler & Co., 1991.

Reputable Suppliers

DeFraine Aromatic Oils
Lavender House,
13 Carlton Road,
Sidcup,
Kent, DA14 6AQ.
Tel. 081–302 1946.

Essential oils, ready-made blends, base oils, white lotion base, pottery essence burners, light-bulb rings, dropper bottles, tea-tree cream and shampoo, etc. Send s.a.e. for details of mail order, retail outlets and courses in aromatherapy, massage and reflexology.

Butterbur and Sage, Ltd.
101 Highgrove Street,
Reading,
Berks, RG1 5EJ.
Tel. 0732 314484.

Essential oils, base oils, tea-tree cream and shampoo, essence burners, books, etc. Send s.a.e. for details of retail outlets and mail order.

About the Author

I discovered the benefits of aromatherapy in 1979 when a counsellor recommended me to try it for a physical and emotional condition I was suffering from. Consequently, I became so intrigued by aromatherapy that I took it up as a career. After approximately 18 months' training with recognised schools I qualified in Massage and Aromatherapy in 1981. Since then I have worked continuously with aromatherapy on a full-time basis in my busy private practice, treating people from all walks of life – from millionaires to housewives.

In 1987, I volunteered my services to a local day centre for severely mentally and physically handicapped young adults. The results were so encouraging I was approached by the local authorities to set up a training programme of elementary aromatherapy for the staff. The training programme has since spread to other organisations for the handicapped and children with special needs.

During my career I have lectured and given courses to a wide variety of groups and societies, including qualified practitioners, in Britain, Israel and the United States. I have been featured in several newspaper and magazine articles both here and abroad, and have spoken on several radio programmes.

Currently I am a consultant for DeFraine Aromatic Oils, Chairperson of the Holistic Aromatherapy Foundation and tutor for the Natural Oils Research Association. I regularly run courses in aromatherapy and massage to diploma level.